Eye Yoga

How you see is how you think

Simple eye exercises to improve your vision
and eye-brain connection

Dr. Jane Rigney Battenberg

Martha M. Rigney

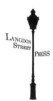

Langdon Street Press
212 3rd Avenue North, Suite 290
Minneapolis, MN 55401
612.455.2293
www.langdonstreetpress.com

ISBN - 978-1-934938-75-1
ISBN - 1-934938-75-0
LCCN - 2010930668

Typeset by James Arneson

Printed in the United States of America

ENDORSEMENTS

"*Eye Yoga* is a visionary book about vision. It offers state-of-the-art practices to improve one's seeing of both outer as well as inner worlds. The authors address both sight and insight in ways that add new possibilities to human experience. The techniques offered here are superb and enhance both physical and mental performance in unexpected and deeply gratifying ways. Read this book, do the exercises and see a new world."

—Jean Houston, Ph.D., author of numerous books including *A Passion for the Possible, A Mythic Life,* and *Jump Time*

"The eyes guide your every move. Thus, your vision is reflected in every step you take. Change your vision and your life will surely change. This book will show you how."

—Jacob Liberman, O.D., Ph.D., author of *Light: Medicine of the Future, Take off Your Glasses and See,* and *Wisdom from an Empty Mind*

"*Eye Yoga* challenges the current myths about vision and gives the reader a very clear road map on how to improve one's eyesight and vision. The exercises are excellent tools to help a variety of vision problems. I highly recommend it!"

—Sam Berne, author of *Creating Your Personal Vision*

"Stated in simple language without hype, *Eye Yoga* is a uniquely gentle path to better vision. It is eager curiosity not forced discipline that brings success. In the process you'll discover how your brain works your eyes to see your deeper self."

—Ray Gottlieb, O.D., Ph.D., author of "Neuropsychology of Myopia"

"This is an excellent book. Just as our vision serves to connect our inner and outer worlds, this book serves to make many important connections for the reader—connecting the eye with the brain, connecting thinking and seeing, and connecting eye exercises with vision. Many of the eye exercises are done with a partner, which serves to create another connection. I highly recommend this book."

—Dr. Neal Apple, Ophthalmologist

"Not only would people with vision problems benefit from reading this book, but so would all psychotherapists."

—Dr. Lee Hartley, Marriage and Family Therapist, Psychotherapist

"You see, you have two miraculous eyes. What they'll learn from reading *Eye Yoga* will reveal the world in all its luminous and beautiful mystery."

—Lance D. Ware, Board-certified hypnotherapist, Somatic Intuitive Training™ Practitioner/Trainer, author, co-founder of ISIS Institute

To our father, Jackson Ashcraft Rigney,
who loved us unconditionally,
who inspired us to be all we could be,
who challenged us to think outside of the box.

This book is for those who are seeking the freedom to see easily, clearly, effortlessly, and enthusiastically all that life has to offer.

A fun
    Effortless
        Insightful
Effective
    Way to
        Influence,
            Improve

My vision
    Physical seeing,
        Awareness of how I see

How I see the world and how I see myself.

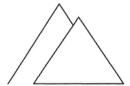

Drink in with your eyes the full spectrum of living
    Including different intensities, tempos,
        Colors and shadows,
            Stillness and movement,
                Detail and overview

To see life's plan
    And life's daily detail,
        Relax and attune
            Into clear vision.

—Martha M. Rigney

WHAT THIS BOOK IS
AND IS NOT / HER-STORIES

What This Book Is

This book is a fun way to help you to achieve improved vision. It requires very simple tools and only a small investment of money and time. It is geared to stretch and relax your eye muscles as well as to educate your eyes and your brain. Many eye problems are linked to tension and stress in the eyes. Our eyes were not made to fixate on computer screens or written pages for long hours at a stretch. The repetitive motion of how we use our eyes on a daily basis can cause strain, just like people who work on assembly lines in factories or tennis players with tennis elbow. If you have ever wanted to try some exercises to relieve that tension and stress in your eyes and brain, you have arrived. You are invited to jump in.

Frequently people find that once they educate their eyes, they do not need to do these exercises as often. Once the eye muscles and brain have been retrained, they seem to remember their new seeing skills and use them all the time. It is possible to continue to improve eyesight in this way.

We use self checks for you to determine your progress results. No need for fancy machines and someone else's evaluation. You can find out for yourself how you are progressing, and you do your own checking whenever you want to.

Are you facing serious eye conditions or diseases? Then you need to consult an eye doctor. Anyone with special problems, diseases, impairments, and disabilities should seek appropriate professional, medical care. This book is not for you right now. Come back once you have received your medical okay.

These exercises should not replace competent optometric or medical care, but should be used as an adjunct to your eye doctor's evaluation.

What This Book Is Not

Vision Therapy is a precise and formal way that eye doctors, primarily behavioral optometrists, treat specific diagnoses. They do a great job with that. But what about those of us who have no serious eye condition and who just want an easy way to educate and evaluate ourselves in order to maintain or improve our vision? With *Eye Yoga* there are no trips to the doctor's office, and the price is right. You don't have a specific diagnosis for an eye problem. You simply do the easy exercises so you can see more clearly with less correction, with occasional use of correction (such as for driving or reading), or with no glasses or lenses at all.

Enjoy This Book

Now relax and find a friend to assist you when you go through the exercises the first time. Enjoy exploring your vision and see how you are wired up. Make friends with your eye-brain connection, so you can use the exercises to their best advantage.

Exercise can be fun while it improves your long-term vision health. We invite you to leave your critic behind and just observe what is happening as you explore the exercises in this book. Enjoy and have a good time with it. Congratulations on choosing this healthy, natural method for improving your vision.

"Not only is keen sight a great convenience, but it reflects a condition of mind which reacts favorably upon all the other senses, upon the general health and upon the mental faculties."

—William H. Bates (Quackenbush, *Better Eyesight Magazine,* July 1920)

HER-STORIES: WHY WE WROTE THIS BOOK

Martha's Story: "Changing my lifestyle dramatically changed my eyesight."

Our family moved to Lima, Peru, when I was in the fourth grade, and my re-entry into the U.S. came in the seventh grade. Shifting cultures once again and trying to find my new place among my peers was a bit confusing, especially at age thirteen. I struggled to see where and how I fit into all this change. I admired my older sister's sophisticated, grown-up look with her new glasses, and soon found myself near-sighted and with glasses. Wearing them was the accepted norm.

I entered the working world after college, and found myself drawn to positions with a lot of focus on the details. First it was international banking operations. Next, I joined IBM, training to be a marketing representative along with fresh college graduates who were first or second in their class. I wanted to do my best. There was great pressure to absorb new material as well as compete with fellow classmates and with myself. After a few years, I took a break from the stressful and competitive marketing environment to do computer programming and manage a data recovery operation for a large insurance brokerage firm. Later, I created a job there as their technical computer-support person, servicing 150 people in three locations. Again, I felt intense time and performance pressures. Finally, something inside me rebelled and I realized: "Life's too short!" So I gave notice and left the pressure-cooker, downtown big-city job.

Over the next few months, I had to stop wearing my contacts, as they were uncomfortable and bothered me too much. I would often resort to wearing my older glasses. Then, even the glasses were a problem. So it was off to the optometrist who told me, "No wonder! Your prescription is way too strong for you." I was astounded that my prescription dropped by about one-third and all I did was remove the stress from my life and not wear my lenses all the time!

Surprised and intrigued, I began my journey into what influences vision. Luckily, my optometrist was a behavioral optometrist who did vision therapy in his office along with color light sessions called Syntonics. The colored lights affect the sympathetic and parasympathetic nervous systems and are soothing or stimulating depending on the color used. I began learning the miracle of what true, healthy vision entails. My journey has been a delightful weaving of vision therapy, color light therapies, natural vision improvement exercises, stress reduction techniques, yoga, nutrition, and mind/thought/body/emotional explorations. Currently, I work with people individually and in groups to explore their visual world. We take a look at their habits, stresses, lifestyle, beliefs, and inflexibilities. Working together, our goal is to expand their awareness to new ways of being and seeing.

Jane's Story: "Changing my eyesight helped me change my lifestyle."

When I turned forty, I married and moved from San Francisco to Orange County in southern California. My cosmopolitan, easy, lifestyle in The City, where I commuted to work on one of San Francisco's famous cable cars, changed instantly. I now had a two-hour commute through congested freeways in addition to my twelve-hour workdays. Coping with corporate budgets, performance targets, and union negotiations was very stressful. Added to this was the need to make new friends and learn to be a wife and step-mom. I developed uncomfortable, itchy skin rashes that spread to my whole body. Enervated, bloated, and unable to sleep, I was uncomfortable in my own skin. As the years passed, I kept increasing the strength of my prescription glasses and became so sensitive to light that I wore dark sunglasses even on cloudy or rainy days. The many drugs and treatments I tried did not stop the condition from worsening.

Eventually, not finding solutions in allopathic medicine, I turned to alternatives such as Neuro-Linguistic Programming's Time Line Therapy©, Vision Therapy, and colored light therapy. Gradually, I began to treat the underlying causes of my discomfort and stress. After sessions of watching a flickering colored light on a machine called a Lumatron, my light sensitivity disappeared, giving me a small, hopeful sign. I began to work with a gifted vision therapist, who showed me that I was unconsciously suppressing vision in my left eye. She explained that it was a metaphor for shutting out everything I couldn't deal with emotionally, as my left eye processed 80% in a right-brained way. One day after a session with her, I began to see with both eyes, seeing the world with depth for the first time. Such a beautiful world opened up! As I continued to work with my eyesight, I taught myself to see farther and to clear up the fuzziness of my vision. Along with the far vision improvement came more ability to cope with the emotional stresses and to envision a more positive future for myself. I worked with the vision exercises until I no longer needed glasses, even passing the DMV eye test.

The most powerful healing came with the emotional therapy. Time Line Therapy© helped me to uncover and change deep emotional patterns that had brought on the distress. At one point, my unconscious mind, communicating via a pendulum, agreed that it would begin the healing process in one month. A month later, I remember waking up and feeling as if the flu had left my body. The recovery process had begun. Gradually the physical symptoms disappeared and my energy returned.

This journey profoundly changed me, like a shamanic death and re-memberment process. Like Persephone returning from the Underworld, I returned with new intuitive abilities and sensitivities. Shedding my old life, I began to reinvent myself, following the glimmering guidance of the Muses of Healing and Service, to learn the nuances and subtleties of emotional empathy as I developed skills in clinical hypnotherapy (my doctorate), Time Dimension Therapy and NLP, Lomilomi Hawaiian bodywork, Reiki, and Huna. Today I see clients and teach. I love my work and am grateful to have seen my way back to health and vitality.

TABLE OF CONTENTS

Foreword   xvii

Acknowledgments   xix

Introduction   xxi

SECTION ONE
Eye Yoga with a Partner and Eye-Brain Connections   1

Chapter 1   Baseline Evaluation   3
Chapter 2   Getting Started   8
Chapter 3   Clock Circles   15
Chapter 4   Figure 8 Stretches   30
                  Using Eye Exercises to Recover from a Stroke   32
Chapter 5   Finger Push-ups   42
Chapter 6   V-In and V-Out   56
Chapter 7   See Circle Variations   65
Chapter 8   Knots on a String   73
Chapter 9   Palming/Sunning   91
Chapter 10 Finishing Up   99

SECTION TWO
Eye-Brain Physiology   107

Chapter 11 Eye-Brain Development   109
Chapter 12 The Vision Process   115
Chapter 13 The Iris as a Reflection or Map   125
Chapter 14 Seeing Eye to Eye   137

SECTION THREE

Seeing and Thinking   141

Chapter 15 Sight and Brain Connection   143
Chapter 16 Personality Traits and the Emotional
Nature of Vision   149
Chapter 17 Factors Affecting Vision   166
Chapter 18 Effects from Visual Intake of Light   183
Chapter 19 Vision as a Metaphor   194
Chapter 20 Form and Function   201

SECTION FOUR

Clearing Blocks to Vision   209

Chapter 21 Emotional Blocks and Limiting Decisions   211
Chapter 22 Background on Time Dimension Therapy   222
Chapter 23 The Process of Time Dimension Therapy   232

SECTION FIVE

Daily Eye Yoga   239

Chapter 24 The Daily Routine   241
Chapter 25 Workout Program   255
Chapter 26 Conclusion—Authors' Note   264

Appendix A Charts   265
Appendix B Personality Tests   272
Appendix C Resources   281
Glossary   294
Bibliography and Suggested Reading   299
Index   310

FOREWORD

There is a proliferation of books claiming that vision function can be trained. Many people, driven by the hope of preventing further deterioration of their eyes, seek out methods for natural vision improvement. Sadly, many humans seek a quick surgical fix or are too lazy to do regular exercises.

It is wonderful to read how the sister team, Martha Rigney and Jane Rigney Battenberg, have pulled the vast array of essentials together in order to give you the best chance to use the *Eye Yoga* concepts. Now you can take care of your eyes in your daily life and have a deep impact on the way you look through them and live in clearness.

For some readers, it may be a new idea that the eyes are controlled by the brain. Let this idea in. Let it sink very deeply. The authors have correctly made this critical connection. You may even go further to the next level of perception, where you discover that the mind directs the brain that in turn controls the eyes.

It is no longer a secret that our eyes are just a biological light gathering device. But, don't be fooled into believing that the light only comes from the outside. There is the human light that, like the nerve impulses that travel down the optic nerve, impacts the function of the retina and the eye. In other words, to see clearly means you, as a human, have to be present through your eyes.

In our modern day living, this is proving more and more difficult. There is much that we may not want to see or be present with. However, the light from within is loaded with many magical chemicals that help one slowly and methodically deal with the traumatic perceptions of our lives. Use the self-help methods so clearly explained in the pages of this book to embark on a wonderful journey of self-discovery, with the potential for more inner and outer clearness.

It is actually about your perceptions. If you examine reality very precisely, the newborn faces a world of relatively meaningless perceptions. *Light* from the world out there comes to the eyes, not some *image* of what is out there! That's right. The only thing that is in the light is coded information. As this light travels through the eye, the optical components alter the form of the information so that you, the human, can better manage to make sense of it all! Actually, the optical components modify the direction and focus of the light to maximize the later interpretive potential of the information. It is this sense-making which is where the real challenge is.

That is not all. The light information arrives at the retina of the eye in an upside-down mode. Yes, that's right. So, from the time your eyes are first opened until your last breath, you will be directing your mind to control your brain to make the right inversion of this upside-down information we call reality.

It is not surprising that each human being's perception can be so different. There are many possible ways to build up an illusionary sense of reality. In addition to the coded light information, we come genetically coded into this world with predisposed perceptual qualities. Martha and Jane correctly show how the iris of the eye carries this code that can be so precisely interpreted.

Now you, as the reader, have the possibility to use cutting-edge information presented in *Eye Yoga* to master how to perceive correctly, and keep your eyes healthy. Do not worry if you forget to do the eye exercises. What is important is to remember who is the symphony conductor of your eyes. It is the deepest part of who you are, your Soul. When you do the eye exercises, remember it is really not about *doing* but more about your *being* with this deepest self as you appreciate the experience of what the exercises bring you. Have fun and enjoy your *Eye Yoga* experience.

Roberto Kaplan O.D., M.Ed., FCOVD
Former Professor of Optometry
Board certified in Vision Therapy
Europe, March 28, 2009

ACKNOWLEDGMENTS

To acknowledge everyone who has influenced and supported us in developing this book would be very long, indeed. However, special thanks to some of the key people must be a part of the book. We owe special thanks to Suzan Wilkerson Dallé for introducing us to vision improvement and the eye-brain connection. We are grateful to our mentors and teachers, Jean Houston, Jacob Liberman, Roberto Kaplan, Ray Gottlieb, Sam Berne, Meir Schneider, Larry Jebrock, and Tad James for encouraging us to write this book as well as sharing their wisdom and giving us broad shoulders they challenged us to stand on.

To friends and family who endured the gestation and birthing pangs of the book with us, we thank Martha's husband Ron Brande, Rich Allen, Karse Simon, Chavanna King, Joanne Martin, and Moriah St. Clair. To our mother, Vie Rigney, we owe the greatest thanks for not only encouraging us from the first writings to the very end, but also for writing her own book at the age of ninety just to show us how! To Dusty White, special thanks for the name, Time Dimension Therapy. Thanks to our editors, Diane Nichols, Lance Ware, and the staff of Mill City Press, who courageously red-lined while preserving the heart and soul of the book. To Kelly Krajacic and Greg Krajacic, we owe gratitude for many late nights in troubleshooting and creating the graphics. Thanks to Celeste Mendelsohn for her illustrations crafted with such artistic skill, and to Lynda Banks for her creativity in designing the book cover.

INTRODUCTION

Your eyes respond to muscle stretching and exercise in many ways, like the rest of your body. Keeping good muscle tone and flexibility in the eyes can help you keep good vision as well as keep your eyes healthy. We have a lot more influence over our vision than many of us may think.

One way to influence good vision is through regular eye exercises and stretches, which we call Eye Yoga. Another way is to understand that how you are seeing is closely connected to your brain functions and thought patterns. Once we learn this, many of us are able to positively influence our vision.

This book is the result of years of personal application to improve our own eyesight as well as working with clients to improve their vision and from many workshops given on the subject. We have tried to keep it simple to encourage you to enfold the techniques into your daily routine, for it is with regular practice that habits are changed and long-term results are achieved.

—The authors

Many of us can improve our vision by doing the Eye Yoga (eye stretches and exercises) in this book. We have selected a few of the many eye exercises available to provide an Eye Yoga routine that is simple, yet effective. They form a daily workout that can be incorporated into most people's busy schedules. Eventually, this will evolve into automatically using our eyes in healthier ways.

Most books that deal with vision improvement only give exercises and relaxation techniques. This is good as far as it goes; however, linking physical vision to brain function provides a broader perspective to facilitate improvement. Seeing is actually controlled and directed by the brain. How you see gives insight into how you think. Improving eyesight therefore affects your brain's capabilities. Improving the communication between your brain and your eyes can also improve your vision. We have two levels going on at once in this book that make it unique—the exercises themselves and the information regarding the eye-brain connection.

Yoga Connection: With the word "yoga" in our title, you may wonder what connection eye exercises have with traditional yoga. The surface connection is with the type of workout, using stretching as well as strengthening, breathing, and communication with the brain's inner vision. The connection actually goes even deeper. Traditional yoga is a system of exercises designed to enlighten the mind, expand consciousness, and stimulate body health. While there are many types of yoga and many meanings for it, one traditional meaning is to unify the body and the mind into a higher consciousness, becoming one with Spirit. Body and mind complement each other like an ideal marriage, sparking and magnetizing each other into wholeness.

Eye Yoga is a system of exercises intended to complement this yogic process by breaking the trance of limiting habits and ideas about vision and consciousness. It is intended to open your eyes to an expanded range of vision and to align your inner and outer vision while promoting healthy eyes. It unifies the physical eyesight with the internal vision, the insight, in an eye-brain connection bringing the two together in a higher consciousness, symbolic of the third eye. The program leads to an expanded sense of awareness, like seeing the three-dimensional space between objects, revealing a vision of all-is-one and everything being connected.

The book is divided into the following sections:

Section One: Before beginning the exercises, you should check your eyes to determine a baseline for your vision. That way you will be able to periodically recheck for vision improvement. You then learn about each of the exercises, including what they are for and how to do them with a partner. Then the eye-brain connection is explained, along with suggestions for ways in which you can personalize the information.

The best way to learn the Eye Yoga exercises and their correspondence to the brain is with a partner. A partner can provide you with feedback about what your eyes are doing. You will soon be able to feel this for yourself. This information will be needed when you do the exercises in your daily Eye Yoga workout. A partner will also be able to give you feedback on your eye-brain connection.

Section Two: This section discusses the physiology of the eyes as an extension of the brain. The anatomy of the eye gives a map, or schemata, of the different parts of the eye. What the eyes and nervous system sense is turned into vision by the brain and mind. Light taken in by the eyes also regulates most of our body's life-sustaining functions, such as hormones, rhythms, activity/rest, growth, reproduction, moods, and health. The irises of the eyes are a window into the body's health conditions as well as into innate, genetic personality predispositions.

Section Three: How you see is how you think; how you think is how you see. Vision can both affect and be affected by our thoughts and feelings. We discuss different personality traits associated with various eye conditions and related case stories about how people see as a metaphor of how they deal with life. The effects of light and the interrelationship of form and function are also explored.

Section Four: A process is given for releasing limiting beliefs and emotional blocks to achieve clear vision and good eyesight. A script for a 10-minute visualization process using Time Dimension Therapy techniques from Neuro-Linguistic Programming (NLP) is provided. An explanation is given for how, by using this process, positive results are possible from quantum, biological, and scientific points of view. The Neuro-Linguistic Programming Model of Reality is explored, showing how we actually create our reality.

Section Five: Vision can be maintained and improved by doing Eye Yoga on a regular basis. After initially doing the exercises with a partner, this section gives a description of how to do each of the exercises on your own. It takes you through exercises that are graduated from easy to difficult, ending with a relaxation, like the cool-down in body yoga. Similar to going to a gym, the only way to get results is by doing the exercises consistently. This section also provides the necessary steps and tools to help you be consistent and motivated, such as a Workout Plan, Exercise Tracking Sheet, and more.

In addition to the above main sections of the book, we have included our personal stories of how we got into this in the first place, a Glossary at the end for easy term definitions, and, finally, a Bibliography for those who want to go into more depth. Appendix A contains a copy of all the charts needed for Eye Yoga. Appendix B contains two self-tests for your personality, which filter what and how you see. Appendix C gives further resources, such as associations that can help you find an eye doctor in your area who understands vision therapy and improving eyesight.

We hope you enjoy this book! We wrote this book to give a simple way to keep your eyes and your brain healthy and functioning well, no matter what age you ripen to be.

We would appreciate any feedback or stories about its use. You may direct feedback to our emails. We are available for individual client work as well as workshops.

Jane Rigney Battenberg
eyeyogajane@gmail.com
changewithin.com

Martha M. Rigney
eyeyogamartha@gmail.com

EYE YOGA WITH A PARTNER AND EYE-BRAIN CONNECTIONS

CHAPTER I

BASELINE EVALUATION

Before starting to do the exercises in the next chapter, we suggest that you check your eyes to get an idea of how you see far away and how you see close up. This will tell you your starting point for your vision improvement. You will then be able to periodically recheck your vision and track your progress.

Now tell the truth: Would you really believe that Eye Yoga could improve your eyesight? Well, like the participants in our workshops, give it a try. First, evaluate your eyesight so you have a baseline. Then, after each exercise, re-check your eyesight to see if it has improved. That way you will know if these exercises are for you. Do the evaluation without contacts or glasses if at all possible.

Using the Far Sight (E) eye chart, such as the one in this chapter, stand a measured distance away and see how many lines down you can read. This measures your distance vision. Note your baseline sight—how far away you were from the chart and how far down the chart you could see. Next, hold the Near Sight Chart a measured distance away and see how many lines down you can read. This measures your sight up close. Note both the distance you held the chart from your eyes and the smallest line number you were able to read.

Once you have evaluated and logged your far- and near-sight measurements, you have a baseline for your own vision. What the measurement happens to be is not as important as the changes in it after you do the Eye Yoga exercises that follow.

Far: How far from the chart?_____

How many lines down could you see?_____

Near: How far away did you hold the paper?_____

How many lines down could you read?_____

During your ongoing routine, record subsequent measurements on the tracking sheet at the end of this chapter.

FAR SIGHT CHART

E

BDR

FXOPTS

ENCWABD

MQFURPSG

AOBLSFDTRM

JDTBFQXZPSGAR

NEAR SIGHT CHART

Now measure your nearsightedness by reading the lines below. How many lines down can you read?

1. I must be a sight for sore eyes! Good site is all in location.

2. Good sight is in the eye of the beholder. Behold how good my sight is, for I am actually reading this.

3. Good sight is in the eye of the beholder. Behold how good my sight is, for I am actually reading this. I must be a sight for sore eyes! Good site is all in location.

4. Good sight is in the eye of the beholder. Behold how good my sight is, for I am actually reading this. I must be a sight for sore eyes! Good site is all in location.

5. Behold how good my sight is, for I am actually reading this. Good sight is in the eye of the beholder. I must be a sight for sore eyes! Good site is all in location.

6. Good sight is in the eye of the beholder. Behold how good my sight is, for I am actually reading this. I must be a sight for sore eyes! Good site is all in location.

7. Good sight is in the eye of the beholder. I must be a sight for sore eyes!   Behold how good my sight is, for I am actually reading this. Good site is all in location.

8. Good sight is in the eye of the beholder. Behold how good my sight is, for I am actually reading this. I must be a sight for sore eyes! Good site is all in location.

9. Good sight is in the eye of the beholder. Behold how good my sight is, for I am actually reading this. I must be a sight for sore eyes! Good site is all in location.

10. Good sight is in the eye of the beholder. Behold how good my sight is, for I am actually reading this. I must be a sight for sore eyes! Good site is all in location.

11. Good sight is in the eye of the beholder. Behold how good my sight is, for I am actually reading this. I must be a sight for sore eyes! Good site is all in location.

12. Good site is all in location. Good sight is in the eye of the beholder. Behold how good my sight is, for I am actually reading this.

EYESIGHT TRACKING SHEET

Date	Far Chart Distance	Far Line Read	Near Chart Distance	Near Line Read	Notes

CHAPTER 2

GETTING STARTED

"Our eyes are like any other part of the body; if we exercise them, they will stay young and flexible."

—Dr. Samuel A. Berne, Optometrist

About Eye Yoga

Vision can be maintained and even improved by doing Eye Yoga. Simply by doing exercises, like going to a gym, you can improve your eyesight. You don't need fancy equipment. With only a few simple exercises, you can start your Eye Yoga program right away. However, just like going to a gym, you need to do it on a regular basis. It isn't very realistic to go once or twice and expect to get fit or lose weight. Eye Yoga needs to be done frequently and to become a lifetime program, just as keeping physically fit does.

This section takes the reader first through a warm-up, then to exercises graduated from easy to difficult. It ends with a relaxation, like the cool-down in body yoga. The exercises are geared to be done with little equipment, and they are designed so that you can do them even during a busy day or at home. While there are many more exercises that can be done, we have chosen these to give you the best results with simplicity.

A seventy-six-year-old man came to our Vision Improvement Workshop to "refresh up" on the Bates Method of vision improvement he had learned and practiced decades ago. Afterwards, he traveled the considerable distance back home, excited to start working toward his goal of a renewed driver's license with no restrictions. A postcard arrived a few months later reporting his success and great pleasure at renewing his license with no restrictions!

"I took Jane's workshop about three years ago and have proven to myself many times how well her eye exercises improve my vision or at least keep it from deteriorating! Whenever I feel my eyesight beginning to slip a little, I am reminded to do those exercises again. It really works because my eyesight gets better once again. If something starts to get fuzzy and I'm too lazy to go find my glasses, I just do those little exercises and it fixes it so I can see."

—D. Enders, Corona del Mar, CA

Relearning Good Vision Habits

Eye Yoga stretches the eye muscles to increase their flexibility, relaxation, ability, and stamina. Since the eye muscles are eight times stronger than they need to be, they don't have to be strengthened so much as stretched, relaxed, and fine-tuned. You will need to balance the eye stretching and strengthening exercises, where the eyes learn to work and see together, with the relaxing, loosening exercises, where you re-pattern your eyes and brain to relax and see.

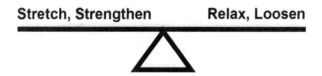

Stretch, Strengthen   **Relax, Loosen**

By moving your eyes in the exercise patterns given, you may be moving them outside your habitual range to give them full extension. In your daily activities, your eyes can get locked into a constricted range of movement, so it is important to stretch them fully. For example, if you habitually don't turn your neck from side to side, you will soon find your neck doesn't turn very well, even when you try. Often the muscles don't know if they are tight or relaxed. In these exercises, you can become aware of tension in your eye muscles and discover what your habitual range of motion is.

Doing Eye Yoga with a Partner

The best way to learn the Eye Yoga exercises and their correspondences to brain functions is with a partner. A partner is needed to give you feedback about what your eyes are doing. You are probably unaware of when your eyes wiggle, when one eye seems to wander or not be engaged, and many other quirky eye movements that don't help clear seeing. With feedback, you will soon be able to feel them for yourself, which is a skill you will need when you do the exercises alone in your daily Eye Yoga workout. In addition, a partner will be able to give you feedback on your eye/brain connections. This feedback is useful to give you insight into how your brain is functioning and how that relates to your vision. This is why we recommend you go through this Eye Yoga section with a partner.

Eye-Brain Connections

We have included the eye-brain connections in with this section for two reasons. First, you have a partner who can help you learn about your unique way of seeing and processing information by observing your eyes to see what you can't notice yourself. Second, it is a more interesting way to learn the exercises by having this additional layer of information inserted where it is relevant. While you are actually doing the exercise, you learn about its connection to brain function. This book is really about how simple eye exercises can reawaken deep brain capacities. We hope you enjoy exploring these ideas and connections!

"Your message is very insightful—the brain can tell the eye what to do!"

—A. Windsor, Newport Beach, CA

"It was such an amazing experience, quite emotional really, to have my brain turn on and off the sight in one of my eyes. I was glad to experience that it really works. All the exercises were so simple yet very effective and profound, especially their connection to right and left brain processing."

— L. F., Costa Mesa, CA

PRE-EXERCISE PREPARATION

Relaxation: As with yoga, you prepare to stretch by relaxing. These five preparations will help the body and the eyes relax and get ready to do the Eye Yoga. They can also be done during the day to take mini-breaks from extended close work or tension build-up. Doing these frequently teaches your eyes the good habits of relaxation, breathing, blinking, and not staring.

- **Breathe:** Inhale deeply and then exhale twice as long, making a sighing sound. As you inhale again (to a count of four), allow the muscles around your eyes, eyelids, even eyebrows to relax. Relax your jaw and your forehead. As you exhale (to a count of eight), let that relaxation ripple down your spine and torso. Breathe again, relaxing your arms and legs. Breathe in and out once more, relaxing your hands and feet.

The eyes use one third as much oxygen as the heart.

- **Blink:** You'd never think of running your car without oil in it. Your eyes need plenty of moisture, so blink your eyes to moisten them. Blinking regularly keeps your eyes healthy as well as keeping you from staring fixedly. William Bates, author and developer of the Bates Method for Better Eyesight Without Glasses, found chronic vision problems arose with habitual unblinking staring. Tense eyelids keep the eyes themselves tense. Blink your lids and you relax your eyes. On an average, we blink about twenty times per minute. Deliberate blinking rests the eyes, massages the eyeballs, and makes the pupils contract and expand. You can consciously blink every three seconds to build up this habit.

- **Twist and Swing:** Looking out horizontally, let your arms and shoulders relax, making them as loose and floppy as possible. Then rhythmically twist your upper torso and head from side to side, letting your arms swing out. Let your eyes also swing freely to the sides, following the movement of your torso without focusing on anything, so the room seems to spin. Do this for about a minute.

Swinging relaxes the body and reprograms natural, smooth, flowing eye movements. It wakes the brain up from a trance of not enough movement and variety in the eye stimulation.

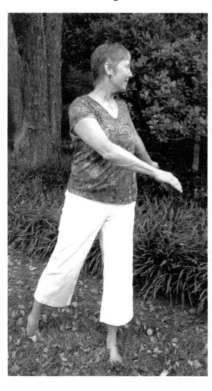 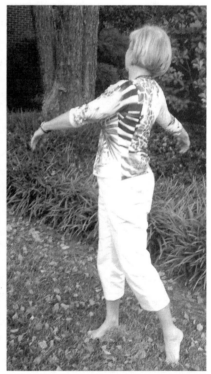

- **Head and Neck Rotations:** Gently roll your head in a circle, first clockwise and then reversed. Relax your neck as much as possible. You may close your eyes for more relaxation. Remember to breathe deeply and slowly.

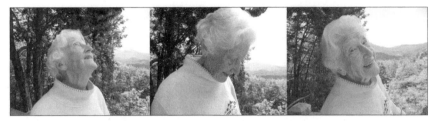

- **Cross Crawl:** As you walk or step in place, raise your right knee and touch it with the palm of your left hand. Then raise your left knee and touch it with the palm of your right hand. Do this ten to twenty times to get the right and left brain in sync.

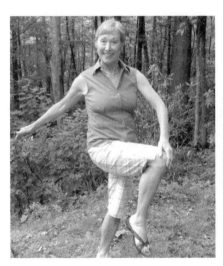

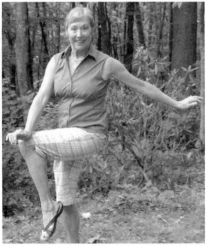

Before starting, you will want to gather a few easy props to use with our simply designed exercises.

Materials Needed In Preparation for Eye Yoga Exercises:

- 6-foot long piece of string or rope with knots tied in it every 8–12 inches
- Copies of pages 5, 6, 7, and 269
  Far Sight Chart
  Near Sight Chart
  Eyesight Tracking Sheet
  See Circles

Now you are ready for Eye Yoga!

CHAPTER 3

CLOCK CIRCLES

STRETCHING WARM-UP

First, you want to gently stretch the muscles around your eyeballs. These are the muscles that turn your eyes in the socket. For a picture of the muscles involved, see the drawing on page 114. You are going to move your eyes slowly around in a circle, starting with your eyes up at a clock's 12:00 position. Keep your head still, not moving it, while your eyes make the circles. Your partner should move their finger slowly around in a circle about 15 inches in front of your face. Watching your partner's finger gives you something to follow. Since you want the eyes to stretch but not strain, help your partner get the circle big enough to provide a stretch but not so big that it is outside of your vision. Help them get the right speed as well so that your eyes are constantly moving at a steady pace but not racing. Pace yourself so that it takes around 10–17 seconds to do one rotation.

12

9

3

6

Partner's Job

- You will want to find the best distance from the exerciser's face so that they can comfortably track your finger. Too far away doesn't stretch the eyes, and too close may be hard to see. Also adjust the size of the circle to be within the range of their vision. You want your finger to always be in the exerciser's field of vision but just at the outside edge of it. Too wide a circle may be beyond where they can see without moving their head. Get the right circle size to give their eyes a nice stretch. Have the exerciser help you make the adjustments.

- Next, adjust the speed of your movement so the exerciser is not racing to keep up, but your movement isn't so slow that they get bored. Go fast enough so that you can see their eyes move but slow enough so they can follow. Instruct the exerciser to try to keep eye movements very smooth as they track your finger.

- Next comes the important part. As you move your finger, watch the exerciser's eyes to see if they are following it. You are looking for zips or jumps and wiggles or glitches. A **zip** is when the exerciser's eye zips ahead to where it thinks your finger is going to go. A **jump** is when an eye suddenly jumps from one position

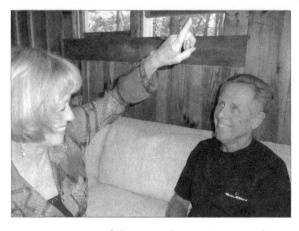

to another, as if pausing, then trying to catch up with your finger, instead of moving at an even pace. A **wiggle or glitch** is when the eye seems to wiggle back and forth with little twitchy micro-movements. Any movement of the eye that is not steady, smooth, and controlled is what you are looking for. Point it out to the person so they can begin to be aware of it and feel it on their own. Do this exercise for a few minutes, until the person begins to feel the stretch and until they can begin to be aware of the zips, jumps, wiggles, and glitches. Almost everyone has these zips and wiggles, however small, so look carefully at the exerciser's eyes to notice them. It may take a bit of practice and observation.

So far, you have had the exerciser practice a gentle stretch, expanding the range of motion of their eyeballs. You have given them feedback on how smoothly they track your finger, pointing out any of the zips, jumps, wiggles, and glitches, so they can begin to feel them themselves. Now let's add another layer to this by talking about which parts of the brain the eyes are accessing in their different positions.

THE EYE-BRAIN CONNECTION

Everything that we take in through our eyes and our other senses gets represented internally in our brain and in our nervous system. We are constantly taking in and processing information both from within ourselves and from the world outside. Since the mind and body make up one interactive, connected system, anything that happens to one, affects the other. Our physical condition affects our thoughts and mood; and, conversely, our thoughts *always* have a corresponding physical reaction. We are continually communicating information about what we are doing internally.

According to Rex Steven Sikes, we use our non-verbal behavior to access different parts of our brain. We use eye movements, head tilts, postures, breathing rates and shifts, arm and hand gestures, skin tone, and qualities of our speech in unique combinations to allow us to access different parts of our brain for processing information. You may have noticed people tilting their heads, taking deep breaths, or looking away when trying to remember something. You may even have used your breath to help you access a calm state, or to think better by taking a slow, deep breath. The type of processing a person is doing is reflected in their many little behaviors.

"It is the unique *combination* of how we sequence movements in the face and body that allow us to access different parts of our brain for processing information."

—Rex Steven Sikes, NLP Mega-Glossary, Accessing Cues (See Dale Kirby's Meta-Web entry in the bibliography)

Conversely, the process of accessing different parts of our brains can be done by consciously using these micro-behaviors. A person can actually learn greater flexibility of thinking and mental processing by adopting different eye movements, facial expressions, head movements, breathing rates, and other body behaviors.

In the movie, *Akeelah and the Bee*, high school student Akeelah would enhance her spelling recall by rhythmically tapping out the rhythm of the word on the side of her leg. Her mentor had her learn new words while jumping rope to a rhythm, to imprint them faster and more firmly in her memory. In one contest, she even mimicked jumping rope so she could get the accurate spelling of a word!

This is what is meant by an interactive process: our thinking affects and is reflected in our body movements and our body movements affect our thinking, with the ability to enhance the thinking process. It is evident that the mind and body are one system with interacting parts. Once this is grasped, it is an easy step to the concept of the eyes and the brain being interconnected parts of the same system.

Eye Patterns

Neuro-Linguistic Programming (NLP) is a series of transpersonal psychology techniques and methodologies formulated in the 1970s by John Grinder and Richard Bandler. They found that the eye positions can access different functions or internal representations in the brain. We actually store and retrieve visual (pictures) when we look up. We store and retrieve auditory (sounds) when we look to the sides, and we access our feelings when we look down.

In Neuro-Linguistic Programming, it was found that people move their eyes into different systematic positions to access and process different senses or **internal representations**, such as visual, auditory, or kinesthetic. Our eyes literally tell what kind of thinking we are doing. Our eyes give clues as to what kind of processing we are doing internally by the direction they habitually look. If the eyes go up, for example, we are remembering or constructing pictures. If they go sideways, we are either remembering or making up sounds. If the eyes go down, we are either paying attention to our feelings or we are talking to ourselves.

AS IF YOU ARE LOOKING AT THE PERSON:

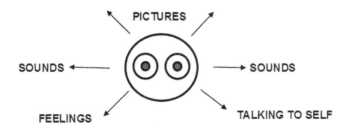

When you want to help yourself access a certain sense, you can move your eyes to a particular position. If you want to remember something you *saw* (visual sense), move your eyes up to recall the picture. How many times have you watched someone move their eyes upward as they were thinking, as if some invisible answer might be written up there? It's as if whatever they are searching for in their brain might be stored there. By moving the eyes upward, they are literally activating the visual aspect of the brain.

If you want to access some sound or remember something that was said, move your eyes sideways. Some people frequently look from side to side, like Richard Nixon used to do when questioned in the Watergate investigation, hence the nickname "Tricky Dick." He was processing the questions and constructing his answers auditorily, which made him appear shifty-eyed.

To remember a feeling, look down. Some people habitually look down, maybe staring off to one side at the floor while talking to another person. As kinesthetic learners, they are processing their feelings at a much slower pace than the zippy visual processors. Watching a person's habitual eye patterns may also give you a clue as to whether they tend to be a visual, auditory, or kinesthetic person. We tend to process information in habitual ways with corresponding personality traits. For a quick test to determine your own primary mode, see Appendix B.

If you ask a person to move their eyes slowly in a pattern, such as the Clock Circles, you may notice that their eye movements are rarely perfectly smooth but usually have zips, jumps, wiggles, and glitches. The ease or difficulty a person has in making these eye movements is indicative of which cognitive and representational processes are habitually more connected or separated for that person. By practicing eye movement patterns such as circles, Zs, triangles, and such, you are linking various parts of your neurology together. You are laying down a physiological path between the different parts of your brain that you use to represent information about the world around you. The ease or difficulty you have in moving your eyes to these different positions indicates the degree to which the neurological pathways are open and smooth. You can get insight into which parts of a person's brain are habitually connected or separated by watching their eyes. You can also tell what kinds of thinking processes a person might excel at or have difficulty with. If, for example, the person's eyes are jerky when looking up, they may be having trouble in the visual area.

Creativity, flexibility, and learning involve the ability to think in different ways. One way to develop new abilities using NLP is to practice various eye movement patterns until they become smooth. Since our eyes reflect patterns of our internal processes, they may be used as a tool for both discovering and for changing habitual thought patterns. Our physiology, in particular our eye movements, forms the underlying circuitry through which we perform our behavioral strategies. Our strategies are only as effective as the neuro-physiological circuitry which supports them.

Creative thinking comes from our ability to link our sensory representational systems together in synesthesias. A *synesthesia* is the cross-linking of senses, where we experience one sense with another. Here are some examples:

—*see* how you *feel* – What is the feeling of that painting?

—*taste* a *color* (visual) – What is the taste of red?

—*hear* the *melody* of a beautiful *sunset* (visual) – What music does the sunset sound like?

—*smell* and *taste fear* (feeling) – What does fear smell and taste like?

—*visualize* and *feel* the *sounds* of a *symphony* – What is the picture of Beethoven's "Symphony No. 9?"

—*hear* the *sound* of his *face* – What is the sound of his face?

—*taste* the *emotions* of this *room* – How do the emotions of this room taste?

Dr. Margaret Mead encouraged people to use multiple sensing at the same time to increase their creativity, problem-solving abilities, and brain capacity. Her remarkable ability to remember and integrate her experiences came out of her tremendous capacity for sensory detail. When we lose this ability to cross-sense, we lose our intelligence. In 1986, Robert Dilts, NLP trainer and author, developed some excellent eye exercises called "Eye Skating: Exercises for the Mind's Eyes," which used eye scanning patterns to explore, enrich, and expand habitual thinking patterns. He says that the process of Eye Movement Desensitization Response (EMDR), developed by Francine Shapiro, employs this type of use of eye movements.

To add a little more to the subject, there is a relationship between eye movements and cognitive processing styles, the way we process, store, and retrieve information. Eye movements seem to trigger the ability to construct (make up) or recall (remember) certain senses. Usually when people look up and to their right (observer's left), they are constructing a new visual image. When they are looking up and to their left (observer's right), they are remembering something they have previously seen.

When they look across to their right, they are creating (constructing) some sound or conversation. When they look sideways to their left, they are remembering something auditory. For most people, feelings are stored down and to their right (observer's left). When they look down and to their left (observer's right), they are analyzing and talking to themselves, an auditory-cognitive function. Occasionally, the entire pattern will be mirror-reversed for a person. But for the purposes of this book and this exercise, all you have to know is that "eyes up" means visual, "eyes sideways" means auditory, and "eyes down" means feeling or talking to oneself (analysis).

Here is a fun exercise to test this. Ask your partner to remember the house where they grew up (visual). Watch their eyes to see if they flicker up to their right (or left) to get that visual image. If nothing happens, ask them to count the number of windows in that house, or ask them the color and make of their family car when they were growing up. For auditory, ask them to remember the sound of their mother's voice, the sound of a favorite pet, or the screech of finger-nails on a blackboard. You can also ask them what they first heard when they woke up this morning. For kinesthetic, ask them to feel what it would be like to slide in between silk sheets or walk barefoot on a wet, sandy beach. You can also ask them to recall a time when they felt a specified emotion. Watch their eye patterns to see where they go for the information. It works best if you can get them to be unselfconscious, allowing their eyes to roam wherever comfortable.

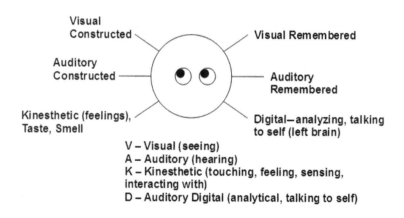

VIEWED AS IF YOU ARE LOOKING AT THE PERSON

Visual Constructed

Visual Remembered

Auditory Constructed

Auditory Remembered

Kinesthetic (feelings), Taste, Smell

Digital—analyzing, talking to self (left brain)

V – Visual (seeing)
A – Auditory (hearing)
K – Kinesthetic (touching, feeling, sensing, interacting with)
D – Auditory Digital (analytical, talking to self)

Strategies are the particular sequence of visual/auditory/kines-thetic/digital patterns a person goes through to retrieve or construct a thought pattern. They are internal strategies followed in order to trigger or elicit certain behaviors. These internal strategies are often given away by a person's eye patterns. For example, when a person goes to buy something, they follow a set sequence. One person may have a sequence of V, K, D, A as a strategy (Visual, Kinesthet-ic, Digital, Auditory). They need to see the items (V), try them on or touch them (K), then make sure the price-to-value is good (D), and finally reassure themselves that they are doing the right thing (A). When you ask them how they bought their watch, their eyes may go up to their left, down right, down left, and then sideways. (More information on this may be found in most books on Neuro-

Linguistic Programming, one in particular being *Frogs into Princes* by Bandler and Grinder).

This information on accessing different senses can be useful in many practical situations. Let's look at the skill used for spelling. If you want to recall how a word is spelled, for example, turn your eyes upward and visualize the word. Practice with the word SUCCESS. Looking up, imagine you are seeing the word SUCCESS above and in front of your face. See the first syllable, SUC, in blue, and the second syllable, CESS, in red. Once you can imagine it, look at the

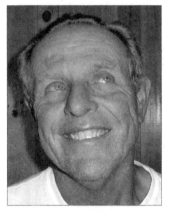

word and read the letters backward, as S S E C in red and C U S in blue. Whenever you need to spell success, look up to "read it."   Teachers often mistakenly tell students who are looking up when asked a question that the answer isn't written up there. In fact, it is!

If you want to memorize something you are studying, place the material higher than your head so you have to look slightly up to study it. That way you are actually placing the material into the visual part of your brain, where it will be when you want to retrieve it. In summary, you can raise your eyes up to either install something into your visual memory or to recall some visual memory.

There is one more use for looking up, that of constructing a picture. If you are an architect or a planner, you may "look up" in order to construct a new design. It is much easier to visually construct when your eyes are raised rather than lowered.

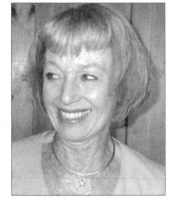

The same use of eye movements may be applied to recalling or constructing sounds (conversations, music, auditory memories, and such).   Sounds and conversations are stored and can be accessed by moving the eyes sideways. In the 2006 Winter Olympics Opening Ceremonies, television cameras showed a young girl singing the Italian national anthem. All the while, her eyes looked from right to left, as she evidently was "constructing and remembering" the sounds of the words and melody of the song.

Feelings and physical sensations, the kinesthetic components, are accessed by looking down. Once I asked a client how she felt about a situation. Her eyes looked up as she told me what she *thought* about it. With my finger, I guided her eyes to look down as I re-asked the question. She said, "Oh, *that*! Well, it makes me feel very sad…" And she launched into describing her feelings instead of her thoughts. Conversely, if a person gets overly emotional and wants to pull out of the inundating feelings, they should move their eyes up. You may have seen someone who is trying not to cry move their eyes way up, as if 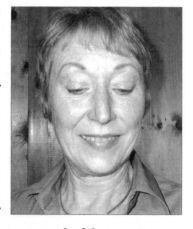 looking skyward, in their struggle to gain control of their emotions. When a client gets sucked down into a negative emotion, I tell them to look up, keep their eyes looking up, maybe even stand up and walk as they do. This invariably pulls them out of the experience of the emotion and into a visual, emotionally detached (dissociated) mode.

Lisa Wake, NLP Trainer, consultant, and psychotherapist in North Yorkshire, U.K., reports she has used eye-accessing exercises to treat children with dyslexia. She modestly suggests that every child that she has used this with has "resolved their dyslexia" (meaning it is no longer manifest). For 60–70% of the children, these exercises were all that was needed to resolve the dyslexia. Another 30–40% required therapeutic metaphor and an adapted form of Time Line Therapy© using games and play.

She designs games that involve each child developing their Visual Construct and Visual Remembered quadrants. The games also disconnect the kinesthetics of negative feelings and self talk from the child's visual processing. Also included are traditional children's games such as "I spy" for visual recall and scribble drawings that encourage Visual Construct. The "number-plate" game is used on car journeys, where the child is encouraged to make up imaginary animals from car number plates. A license plate TP34ENY might become "tiny pointed-ear namby yak." Then the child describes that animal. "Trucks" also involves a car journey game, where the child spots a truck and then describes what she or he imagines to be inside of it. For example, a Walmart truck is imagined to contain rows of shelves with candies, tissue paper, and cookies. In Lisa's experience, one or both parents may also have limited use of the visual quadrants, so these games also encourage development of visual processing in the parent.

Clock Circles Exercise

You may be wondering, "What does all of this mean to me?" It means that you may get a little more insight into your own way of processing information, whether in pictures, sounds, or feelings. You may wonder why the eyes sometimes have trouble moving smoothly around in a circle, and what that has to do with accessing different senses and functions in the brain. It may be linked to your ability or desire to access that part of your brain. If you tend to zip over or have jerky eye movements in the visual area, it could indicate some trauma you saw in your life. Maybe there was something you don't particularly want to remember visually. Maybe you just got lazy visually, or perhaps you do this out of habit. If the eye movement is not smooth when transitioning to the feeling area, perhaps the person is not used to accessing their feelings. It could be a result of anything from a highly emotionally charged event, to an inconsequential thing, maybe a minor habit. We don't always know what is actually going on, and it isn't important. What is important is to know that when you practice, you can smooth out the zips and wiggles.

Smoother eye movements allow your brain to access the different functions more easily. Who cares if it was a trauma, if you can fix it? It's like the chickens who all laid their eggs, except one chicken. She tried and tried, and finally in the afternoon she laid her egg. She cackled and went off to get something to eat. That's it. Who cares why she didn't lay her egg quickly? She didn't sit down to analyze why she had trouble. She just went off to get something to eat. If you smooth the movements out by practicing the eye rotations, thereby eliminating the zips and wiggles, you can increase your brain's ability to access that part and function of your brain more easily. In this way, you increase your creativity as well as your brain's processing faculty.

In summary, by doing these simple eye exercises, you can increase your ability to access these different internal representations: the visual, the auditory and the kinesthetic. You can make it easier to construct or remember visually and auditorily. You can more easily get in touch with feelings and sensations. The exercises also help you to move more smoothly from one sense to another, from visual to auditory, for example. You can increase your skill in using these internal representations in your daily life merely by smoothing out your eye movements. An eye exercise that helps us in these areas can have great value, as these abilities are very closely linked to our creativity and to our mental facility. In this sense, you are also "exercising your brain."

BACK TO CLOCK CIRCLES

Giving Feedback to Your Partner

The partner who is moving their finger around in the circles and giving feedback to the exerciser concerning zips and wiggles, can now give feedback on the areas where the person is having trouble. For example, you may say, "You seem to be having some erratic wiggles up in the visual area" or "When you move your eyes down into the feeling area, they tend to get jerky." As you point it out, you can rotate your finger back and forth in the area where the person is not smooth, so they can experience the jerkiness as well as practice getting smoother movements. You might even make a note for the person as a reminder when they do their daily Eye Yoga exercises. Draw a circle on a piece of paper to note where the zips and wiggles are and whether they are in visual, auditory or kinesthetic areas. Note the smoothness of the transitions between the areas, such as between visual and auditory or from feeling to visual. Be sure to let your partner know when they have gained smoothness!

Palming—Exercise Completion

After doing this exercise for several minutes, feeling the stretch and having begun to sense the zips, jumps, wiggles and glitches, the exerciser should relax and rest the eyes. Rub your hands together to create a little friction and warmth. Then cup your palms gently over your closed eyes, warming them and blocking out all the light. This is called "palming." Quietly take deep, slow breaths and relax your eyes. Let go and deeply relax. Note: Do not press on the eyeballs, either with your palms or fingertips when doing this relaxation.

Check Your Vision

Now just for fun, re-check your vision to see if there has been any improvement at all. Frequently, people will immediately see a slight improvement. It is encouraging to see that a small amount of eye stretching can relax the eyes into better vision. If you do not notice any improvement, don't worry. Sometimes the eyes tire when doing something unfamiliar or that is a "stretch." Remember the gym—it doesn't all happen at once.

Daily Eye Yoga Exercise

After initially doing this with a partner, you are ready to do this each day on your own. Begin your yoga routine with the Clock Circles exercise. Use your own finger to make the circles, so your eyes have something to track.

If you want to deepen the relaxation during the exercise, you may try this "tennis-ball-on-a-string" variation. Attach the string to something like a ceiling fan, lamp or doorway so you can lie down with your face right underneath the tennis ball, close enough so you can reach the ball to swing it. Push the tennis ball in a circle and follow it with your eyes, while holding your head still. Then reverse the direction of the swing. Have the ball also move from side to side in vertical, horizontal and diagonal patterns. Your eyes are free to follow the ball without having to move your finger, a much more relaxing way to do this exercise.

CHAPTER 4

FIGURE 8 STRETCHES

A variation of the Clock Circles exercise is to move your eyes slowly in Figure 8 patterns. At first you may want to use your finger to track the Figure 8, but the finger is not necessary once you get the hang of it. The Figure 8 is easier than the Clock Circles to do during a busy day "on the fly," as it were, or whenever you have a minute to stretch your eyes. Because you don't need to use your finger, it is also less conspicuous.

Partner's Job

Move your finger in a slow, horizontal Figure 8 pattern. Then move it in a vertical Figure 8. Your finger gives your partner something to focus on as they move their eyes in this pattern. Eventually, they will be able to use their own finger or do it without a finger to focus on. Give your partner feedback on zips and wiggles.

Figure 8s

1. Horizontal Figure 8s: Without moving the head, follow your partner's finger as it moves slowly in a Figure 8 motion.

Figure 8 Stretches

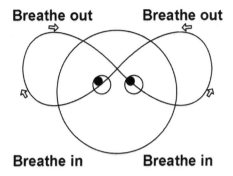

Breathing: Breathe in as you look from down left to up left, and breathe out as you look from up left to down right. Then breathe in from down right to up right and breathe out from up right to down left. Continue this breathing pattern smoothly and easily.

2. Vertical Figure 8s: Start by looking straight ahead at your partner's finger. Following their finger, your eyes will circle out and up to the right, circle around to up left and back to center. Circle eyes down right and around to down left and then back to center. Repeat 8 times or less if your eyes begin to feel tired.

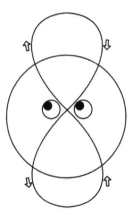

Breathing: Breathe in and out once with each half of the 8, as you did above. Move your eyes as slowly and smoothly as possible in a continuum, instead of jumping from one spot to another.

OTHER BENEFITS FROM CLOCK CIRCLES AND FIGURE 8 STRETCHES

In addition to general stretching, these stretches seem to be particularly good for reducing *astigmatism*, where the muscles are pulling unevenly on the cornea, causing it to warp or wrinkle (see Glossary). Stretching and deep breathing help to relax the tight eye muscles that pull on the cornea and "wrinkle" it.

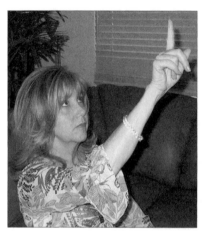

"When I did these exercises in the workshop, I was <u>not</u> comfortable at all looking up. It made me feel dizzy and uncomfortable. My eyes wiggled around and wanted to avoid looking there. Within less than a week, that all went away and I felt confident and comfortable doing the exercise! I was amazed at how quickly my eyes became accustomed to the movements."

— J. Sinclair, Laguna Beach, CA

Using Eye Exercises to Recover from a Stroke

As we were preparing this book for publication, a friend shared the following story of how he used simple eye exercises and visualizations to recover from a severe stroke.

"I woke up at 4 a.m. and thought I'd just slept too long on my left arm that felt asleep, so I wiggled my body around to get the feeling back and went back to sleep. I woke up again around 7:30 a.m. in a hot sweat. I was so hot that I thought something must be wrong. When I couldn't sit up, I noticed that my tongue felt very fat. Then I realized my whole face was numb. I could move my right arm and leg but nothing on my left side. When I touched the left side of my face, it was numb. I couldn't talk—no words would come out—just sounds with no clarity. I lay there

Figure 8 Stretches

for a time with no idea what to do. Then I heard my NLP trainer's voice in my head explaining that when people go into trauma, their eyes stare straight ahead fixedly. I remembered him saying it is important to get their eyes moving around in all quadrants of their head. If there is an injury to the brain it will cut down the time it takes to recover from the injury. By moving the eyes in circles or figure 8s, the person will access the visual, auditory and kinesthetic areas of their brain.

"I began to try moving my eyes up and down in a lazy eight pattern. At first I couldn't move my eyes to the left. After doing the eye movements for a time, I began the process of thinking what to do and of beginning to move to try to get help. It took me 40 minutes to sit up, which totally exhausted me. My tongue was hanging out the side of my face and I still couldn't speak. How was I going to ask for help even if I could get to the phone? I fell onto the floor and struggled for about an hour to move the 8 feet to the door and another hour to get the 12 feet to the phone. As I was lying on the floor panting between my wiggling struggles to move, I again repeatedly did the eye tracking exercises.

"During this two-hour ordeal to get to the phone, I moved my eyes to Visual Remembered and remembered seeing myself in the mirror talking, remembering the sounds my voice made as I talked, recalling how it felt to talk and move. I remembered how to spell the words "I need help," and I remembered the sounds of each word. I practiced over and over in my mind visualizing, hearing and feeling myself saying, "I need help." I practiced making the sounds of "I need help" until I thought I could be understood, at which time I dialed my friend. I said, "I– need– help," and when he asked what was wrong, I kept repeating, "I need help." He called 9-1-1 and they got me to the hospital, where I was diagnosed as having had a stroke.

"In recovery they told me that everyone is different, but the size of the hemorrhage was pretty big. My kidneys were damaged, and it was lucky I didn't die. Generally people with that kind of a stroke take two years to be able to walk. Many can get gross movement within a year. They warned me not to expect to walk for quite awhile, for sure not in the three months I was there. While I was there, I would do my eye exercises every day, staring at the ceiling, doing the sideways Figure 8s. I would also move my eyes in a box and diagonally from up to down. I was literally rewiring and rerouting my brain to create different pathways so the messages could go to the left side of my body. For two months I had no response from my left side, and my tongue was hanging out of the left side of my mouth. When they would move my body, I would do the eye exercises, remembering what it felt like to move, visualizing myself doing the movements. At two and a half months, I began to move. They let me have my first go with a cane. As I walked, I moved my eyes up to Visual Remembered to visualize how I remembered seeing myself and other people walk. I would look down to Kinesthetic to feel how good it used to feel to walk. The end result was that at three months I walked out of the hospital!

"While I was in the hospital, there was another patient who had also had a stroke. He had made no progress in the six months he was there. He was well into his eighties, so they didn't seem to give him as much attention, possibly thinking he would be in long-term care for the rest of his life. So I taught him the eye-tracking exercises as well. As I explained to him what I was doing, he also began doing the eye-trackings. Soon he, too, began to walk, and he was also released. Even though eye-tracking exercises are not standard procedure for stroke recovery, I wish physical therapists would be open to using this, since it helped both of us so much."

—R. Hunt, NLP Trainer, B.C., Canada, rdhunt@dccnet.com

As it happened, I was fortunate to be able to further test the effectiveness of the eye-pattern exercises in combination with visualizations and imaginal body work as this book was going to press. While on

Figure 8 Stretches

a two-week trip around Egypt with Dr. Jean Houston, we were joined by the chairman of Quest Tours, Mr. Mohamed Nazmy. He was recovering from a stroke he'd suffered six months earlier, which had left his right side quite impaired. He walked with a cane, swinging his right leg forward from the hip to take a step, and his right arm was weak with limited movement. Dr. Jean Houston, her assistant Peggy Rubin and I worked with Mohamed during our Nile cruise to create new psycho-neural pathways in the brain for him. Our work included Figure 8 eye/tongue exercises, envisioning using right-left brained multisensorial repatterning and real and imaginal body work. Mohamed, encouraged by improvements in his walking, movement and balance, invited me to stay on an extra eight days as his guest to continue the work. Excited about the prospect to further test the eye-brain connection through our eye exercises, I readily accepted.

We worked every day for two to four sessions, lasting from 10 minutes to 2½ hours. They always included the basic eye exercises of Clock Circles and Figure 8s while moving his tongue in the opposite direction (e.g., eyes circle clockwise while tongue circles counter-clockwise). This went along with imaginal and real body exercises taken from Jean's work and mentioned in section 3, chapter 17, Visual Imagery. For example, he would move his left leg while imagining moving his right leg. Then he would move his right leg while imagining moving his left. He would move both legs while imagining his right side was moving as smoothly as the left.

Visualizations became a powerful core of our work. As Mohamed moved his eyes around the visual, auditory and kinesthetic remembered side, he would recall a time in the past when he enjoyed optimal health or when he was doing something physically enjoyable (playing ping pong, dancing, feeling strong at age thirty-five) and envisioning his body moving easily, smoothly and automatically. Then as he moved his eyes around the constructed side, he would envision himself moving easily with strength, saying to himself how quickly and completely he had recovered, experiencing how good it feels to be healthy with full movement restored to his body. Getting his eyes to move in one direction while his tongue moved in opposition was the source of much hilarity, especially when adding other cross-lateral body movements! It was a bit like patting your head and rubbing your stomach. He would also lace the fingers of his two hands together and feel the movement in his right arm as he used his left arm to move and re-teach it.

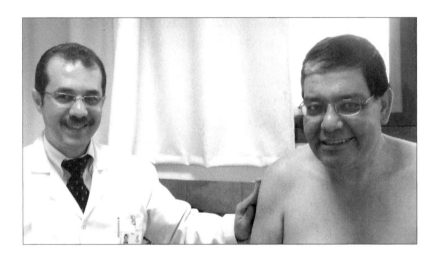

After only two weeks of work, his physical therapy doctors were quite amazed. He used his cane less, often taking stair steps two at a time. The clenched stiffness in his arm and leg were much reduced, as he had learned to send messages to them to relax. New arm and leg movements appeared and his balance was much better. At his last P.T. session he graduated from minimal exercises on the massage table to the large exercise room, where he performed a variety of new movements, including stepping over raised bars, kneeling on a mat and then getting back up, and doing sit-ups. People who spoke with him regularly by phone mentioned dramatic improvements in not only his speech but his thinking. Overall, he achieved a 40–50% improvement in about two weeks.

Upon returning from Egypt, I visited a friend who had had a stroke about six weeks earlier. Due to impairment in his vision, his driver's license had been suspended. I worked with him for about an hour. We did the Figure 8 and Clock Circle eye exercises, adding tongue

Figure 8 Stretches

movements in the opposite direction. He did the cross-crawl exercise while moving his eyes in Figure 8s. Then as he did the circles in the Remembered direction, he remembered a time when he was in the prime of life, including what he looked like, what he said to himself, how he felt. He remembered being on the wrestling team and his girlfriend at the time. As he moved his eyes over to the Constructed side, he visualized himself being able to see, driving well, working in a new way with less stress, experiencing how great it felt to be so healthy and relaxed. Then back to the Remembered side, visual, auditory and feeling memories, before returning to the Constructed side where he built how he would look, feel and talk to himself with perfect health. As he performed these visualizations with the circles, he moved his tongue in the opposite direction.

We then did some spine movements with accompanying eye Figure 8s and Clock Circles, also engaging his tongue and head in opposite directions. He lay on the floor with his knees bent, slowly moving the knees from one side to another as he moved his head in the opposite direction while doing Figure 8s with his eyes. I also had him imagine being in touch with his "higher self," who merged with him to assist in the repatterning of his brain and body, so that not only his physical body was engaged, but his psychological, metaphoric and spiritual levels were employed as well.

"When I had a stroke about six weeks ago, they took away my driver's license because of my impaired vision. My peripheral vision has come back, but I haven't been able to see between around 6:30 and 12 o'clock on my left side. There was a blind spot that caused half of a person's face to disappear, and I saw flashing lights. After working with Jane for a little over an hour, I had a dramatic change in my vision. The blind spot was reduced by over two thirds. There is still a blind spot between 11 and 12 o'clock, with some flashing, but I can actually see through the flashing instead of it being blank. The improvement has lasted, and after a subsequent phone session a week later, I found the blind spot not only diminished further in size but had also receded to above a person's face with even less flashing.

"There were several amazing things in the work we did. I couldn't see Jane's hand when she held it up, so she told me to move my tongue around. Then I could see it again! I was also surprised that she could tell by watching my eyes when I could see. As an engineer, I find the idea of the brain being holographic to be a very interesting concept in repatterning and healing from the stroke damage."

—Alan Glas, San Anselmo, CA
December, 2008

I had one more opportunity to work with a man in his late fifties who was recovering from a stroke. He used a cane and wanted to walk without dragging his left foot. We worked together for a little over an hour, during which he not only corrected the foot drag but actually was able to run. I asked him if he could run, and he replied that he could not. When I asked him if he was able to jog before the stroke he said yes. After visualizing himself running like before and doing the eye exercises, he could actually jog the length of the room! This gave him encouragement and lifted his mood considerably. In the ensuing days, a close friend commented that his speech and thinking had greatly improved as well. Following is Tony's testimonial:

"I had an inspiring therapy session that was very beneficial in the process of my recovery from a stroke. One of the things that I got out of the therapy session was the prompt to remember what it felt like to walk correctly, and to run with the agility that I did before I had a stroke. The other important lesson was to remember the balance that is needed. With assistance, I was able to attempt things that I had not known that I could do, mainly because I had been restricted to using my cane, walker and wheelchair during the process of recovery. I always wondered whether I could actually walk or even run as I could before the stroke.

Figure 8 Stretches

"The self-hypnosis we did helped to reassure me that I could do these things. It was also helpful to stimulate my imagination, which has always been strong. This meant that I could perceive myself doing something first. From there it was not very difficult for me to actually do the very thing I imagined, like actually running. This was completely consistent with the personal self-hypnosis and relaxation techniques I have been using since my release from intensive care and suggested by my neuro-psychologist. The techniques of self-suggestion are extremely powerful in the process of stroke recovery. Seeing yourself do something and telling yourself you could do it are the two most important parts of accomplishing anything. Remembering how to do it calls to the fore remembrance of all the necessary machinations, actions, movements and processes. As they say on the street, 'There's nothing left but to do it.'

"The various exercises involved eye, tongue and head movements. I am sure they are helpful in the process of re-establishing neural pathways and remapping the brain. I previously attended a seminar on this subject. But what was missing were exercises to actually accomplish this. These exercises seem to do exactly that.

"As I came away from the session, I began to ask myself what other types of multitasking I could consider attempting. The phrase, 'If you don't use it, you'll lose it' is one of the most important for the stroke victim to remember. If these sessions can reawaken areas of the brain that could become underutilized due to inaction and lack of activity, then the results could be nothing but positive and helpful.

"We must continually challenge our capacities to make sure that we are not telling ourselves that we can't do things that we have not attempted, or forgotten how to do. I myself sat in a bed in intensive care following the stroke wondering if I could actually walk. From the level of physical therapy they offered me I assumed that my problem was serious. But they could never give me information about a clear path to 100% recovery. I assumed that I would be confined to the use of a cane, walker and wheelchair from then on. I now believe that it will be possible for me to walk and run and dance as I had prior to the stroke.

"Another important factor in my session was the confidence by all concerned that I got. Keeping a positive state of mind, daily exercise, physical therapy and challenging routines are key elements to recovery. The inspiration of advocates and associates are also essential in this process. I think it is important to let those helping me know about my desire to perform at a higher level and my working hard to recover is vital."

—Tony Fleming, San Francisco, CA
January 25, 2009

In looking for scientific corroborations for our work, I was led into the area of brain neuroplasticity. One of the leading researchers on brain plasticity is Michael Merzenich, who realized that our brains are not hardwired systems but rather plastic in nature. He has developed many ways to improve people's ability to think and perceive, by training specific brain processing areas he calls brain maps to make them do more mental work. He believes "... that plasticity exists from the cradle to the grave; and that radical improvements in cognitive functioning – how we learn, think, perceive, and remember – are possible even in the elderly." (Doidge, p. 46) Merzenich claims we can change the very structure of our brain and increase our capacity to learn because our brain is constantly changing and adapting itself.

Paul Bach-y-Rita, one of the pioneers in brain plasticity, tells the story of his own father's stroke at sixty-five, which left him paralyzed on one half of his body and unable to speak. Paul's brother George, a medical student, worked persistently with his Catalan poet father, first teaching him to crawl, propping him up against the wall on his weak side for support. He designed exercises and games

Figure 8 Stretches

to work with the weak side. After months he was able to sit up and eat, to walk and even his speech began coming back. At the end of a year his recovery was complete enough for him to resume full-time teaching at City College in New York. He went on to remarry, work, hike, and travel for another seven years. When he had a heart attack at age seventy-two, the autopsy revealed that the parts of the brain that control movement, mainly the brain stem, had been destroyed by the stroke. Somehow his brain had totally reorganized itself to shift normal functioning to other parts of the brain!

Michael Lavery, an artist in Laguna Beach, California, has developed a program to increase brain power, thicken the myelin sheath around the neurons and keep us younger. He has worked with a variety of people, including athletes, professors and medical doctors, to teach them his self-designed methods for improving athletic performance and mental acuity. His methods include mirror-image writing, like Leonardo da Vinci used in his journals, and bouncing ping pong balls off hefty ball-peen hammers, switching hands, while reciting the numbers of pi. He says the secrets are in using the hands, eye-hand coordination and ambidextrous exercises while performing mental gymnastics.

CHAPTER 5

FINGER PUSH-UPS

In this exercise you are practicing what is called converging, having both of your eyes turn in and out evenly, working together. This also helps to increase flexibility and relaxation, increasing the eyes' range of motion. It is particularly good for those who have trouble seeing things up close and for those who need or are beginning to need reading glasses.

Start with a few deep breaths. Relax while you imagine the oxygen going to your eyes. Then your partner will hold their index finger out in front of you, about two to three feet away from your nose. Focus on the tip of their finger. Continue watching it as they slowly bring their finger in toward the tip of your nose and back out again. As you do this, notice any stretching sensation in your eyes. Keep the tip of their finger in focus as much as possible. Repeat this slow in-out movement for five to eight times. Then, cup your palms over your closed eyes and relax them. You may be able to feel that your eyes have been exercised. (For the record, it is an old wives' tale that your eyes can get stuck by "crossing them." Kaplan, *Conscious Seeing*, p. 196)

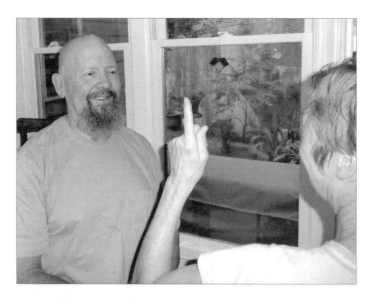

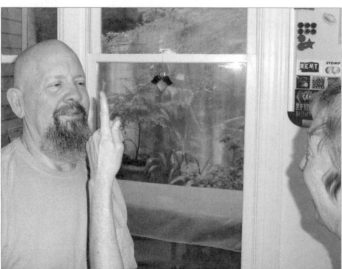

Partner's Job

- Have your partner focus on the tip of your index finger, held several feet out in front of the tip of their nose. Tell them to keep your finger in focus as you slowly move your finger in toward the tip of their nose. If they lose focus, back up and move in more slowly, while they attempt to keep the focus.

- Adjust the speed of your movement so their eye movements are uniform and smooth as they follow your finger. If you move too fast, they won't get the nice, even stretch, and, if you move too slowly, it will be boring.

- Once you have adjusted the speed and range of your finger movement for optimal exercise, your job is to watch your partner's eyes closely and to give them feedback. You are looking to see if both eyes are working together, turning in and out at the same rate. You are also looking for any jumps or glitches. Watch for any differences between the two eyes, such as jerkiness, less movement in one eye, eyes moving back and forth as if trying to decide which one will focus on the target, rapid wiggles or spaciness where an eye doesn't seem to move in or out at all. You may notice one eye giving up and continuing to look straight ahead rather than moving in.

- Give the person feedback, such as:

"Your left eye doesn't seem to be moving or watching my finger as well as the right eye."

"When I get to about here, both eyes seem to stop moving."

"Can you feel your right eye jump right here?"

The differences can be quite subtle, and it may take you a few times to notice them. Often one eye moves better than the other. Identify which eye is smoother, which eye seems to track better. Sometimes the person may seem to be deciding which eye will look at the target, as if they won't look with both eyes at the same time.

If the person has one eye that is less active or less smooth, merely tell that eye to see—to "wake up and work better." Give your partner feedback on any improvement.

If one eye continues to have a problem, cover the other eye and do some Finger Push-Ups with that eye alone. This will give it the experience of doing it on its own rather than relying on the other eye to do more of the work. Then return to using both eyes to see if there is any improvement. Repeat this several times if necessary to get both eyes to work together. It takes practice, and you are not only training their eyes to work in sync, you are also training the person to be aware of when their eyes are working together and when they are not.

- Be sure to stop if the person's eyes begin to tire. It is easy to overdo this exercise. In fact, eye exercises can make the whole body feel tired. As with any new exercise, you do not want to strain the muscles or push beyond what is comfortable.

THE EYE-BRAIN CONNECTION

Right Brain Versus Left Brain Functions

Our brain is made up of two halves, a left brain and a right brain. It is well known that the brain's right hemisphere processes information differently than the left hemisphere. The right brain, associated with the left side of the body, is responsible for orientation in space, artistry, synthesis, face recognition and emotions. The left brain, associated with the right side of the body, is responsible for logic, analysis, language, mathematics, sequence and order.

Right Brain	Left Brain
Emotions, sensuality	Logic, numbers, letters, words
Pictures, faces, places, objects	Words, language, speech, verbal expression
Passion, dreams	Analysis, dissection
Wholes and relationship of parts	Sequential, linear thinking, reason
Synthesis, integrates many inputs simultaneously	Wordsmithing, engineering
(W)holistic, intuitive thinking	Detail-oriented, factual, knows objects
Big picture, makes meaning, sense	Factual science, comprehension
Time-free, can lose sense of time	Sense of time and relationship to goals
Present and future time	Present and past time
Creativity, imagination, possibility	Order, rules
Makes strategies	Objective, direct, blunt
Patterns, context	Specific content
Spatial awareness	Puritanical work ethics, productivity, no pain no gain
Music, artistry, craftsmanship	Earthly, mechanical, material, chemical
Philosophy, religion, believing	Detached intellectual perspective, calculating
Risk taking, impetuous	Practical, safe
Videos, playing, dance, group work, sound, rhythm	Research, individual work, near-point work
Implicit, tacit, gestalt	Explicit, linear
Timeless, eternity	Time, history
Spatial and kinesthetic orientation	Fine motor skills, fine-tuning
Integrates visual, muscular and kinesthetic cues quickly	Fight or flight, type A

Right Brain	Left Brain
Depth perception	Seeing clearly up close
Passive, yielding, cooperative	Judgmental, anchored, grounded
Artistic, images, color, feelings	Math, numbers, computers, symbols, money, digital, segmented, bit-by-bit
Choice, subjective, indirect, subtle, nuances, finesse, shades of gray	Black and white, absolutes, all or nothing
Sees distance clearly, open, divergent, extrovert, outward	Focal information processing, pinpoint, inward, introvert, zeroing in, attention to detail
Seeing the forest and the trees	Seeing the trees for the forest
Presight	Hindsight
Health, relaxation, not run by time	How long will it take, fast-paced, impatient, time is money, speed, bottom-line profit
Putting together	Taking apart
Learning new things	Automatic habits
Initiating	Concluding

These hemispheric differences were first discovered by Roger Sperry and Ronald Meyers in 1963. The two halves of our brain are divided by a big, thick fold called the corpus callosum that goes from front to back in our brain. They are connected to each other by a thick cord of nerves at the base of each brain half. Sperry found that when a cat had its corpus callosum (connection between the two brain halves) and optic chiasm severed, it showed two independent learning centers, one in each hemisphere. If the cat learned a response with its right eye open and left eye covered, it was unable to repeat that response with the left eye open and right eye closed. Sperry concluded that the brain had two separate realms of conscious awareness and two sensing, perceiving, thinking and remembering systems, for which he won the Nobel Prize in Medicine in 1981.

Today this information has spread its applicability to many diverse fields, including psychiatry. Dr. Fred Schiffer, a psychiatrist on the faculty at Harvard Medical School, has found that each side of our brain possesses an autonomous, distinct personality with its own set of memories, motivations and behaviors. Emotional troubles or traumas stored in the brain can be awakened and released by using a special form of visual stimulation to one side of the patient's brain.

"The main theme to emerge... is that there appear to be two modes of thinking, verbal and nonverbal, represented rather separately in left and right hemispheres respectively and that our education system, as well as science in general, tends to neglect the nonverbal form of intellect. What it comes down to is that modern society discriminates against the right hemisphere."

— Roger Sperry (1973)

More recent studies show that humans have a more duplex-operating system, where there seems to be some crossover between the two halves. The two halves can complement each other and work together in their differences. Where the left brain "does," the right brain "is." Each side has different mental organization and functioning skills and each is essential to a complete understanding of the world as we perceive it, perhaps even for our survival. Einstein called it "combinatory play" (Ornstein, p. 36). Many scientific ideas have come on suddenly when the rational, left-brain processes were shut down.

The two halves of our brains see the world in very opposite ways. Even in our society, the left, rational side tends to dismiss anything significant from the right side as being flaky and weird. The left dismisses the arts as "fluff" in education. When considering economic cutbacks, it desires to get back to the basic three Rs and cut out the arts. One can readily see in this War of the Brains where the left brain has dominated in society. Leonard Shlain in *The Alphabet Versus the Goddess* suggests that the left-brained, male-dominant tendency in the world began with the written word, which emphasized the left-brain's functions. In our current society, where television, cinema and DVDs present the brain with multiple, synthesized pictures often in rapid-fire shifts, our children may be developing their right-brain hemisphere to a much greater degree. This may ultimately make a huge shift in society.

Even though both sides of the brain have independent, different functions, we can benefit from the integration of these two types of information processing. It is possible that most people don't reach their maximum potential because of compromises that have been made between the two brains. Sometimes, endeavors which the right brain can undertake better are routinely handled with less skill by the left. Ideally, both brains should work together for optimum mental, emotional and physical abilities and for superior intellectual abilities. The hemisphere best suited to perform the processing will step up to do it, allowing greater understanding of the situation and learning to result.

Even memory works better when both sides of the brain are used. If you need to memorize a list of items in their exact order, the left brain would number each item and repeat the list over and over to memorize it. After about 30 minutes, you will have memorized four or five items on the average. Engaging your right brain in the process as well adds creativity and imagination. Use color, action, pictures and maybe even make up a story using the seven items. This uses the whole brain, and usually results in remembering the items in their exact order for a long time. In fact, it may be hard to forget them, even if you try!

Jacob Liberman, in his book, *Take Off Your Glasses and See* (p. 185), says: "According to a model of brain function developed by psychiatrist, William Gray, and systems scientist, Paul LaViolette, 'the brain uses feelings to structure information. A felt sense underlies everything we know.... When we are cut off from our feeling tones, mental connections become difficult. That is why abstract information is so hard to recall....' This model, which has been supported by several research studies, confirms that the best way to process *any* new information is open thinking, which allows us to access both thoughts and feelings simultaneously."

The right/left brain specialization has received some emphatic criticism, dismissing the idea of a rigid divide or such a thing as a left-brained or right-brained person. While the underlying science of brain specialization of Sperry and others seems to hold, the brain is too complex to be simplified into rigid categorizations. One may learn a task with predominantly left-brain functions (to drive a car) and then move it over to automatic, where we drive almost unconsciously without thinking about every move (a more right-brain domain). As we gain abstraction, information may be passed from one side to another. And one shouldn't forget the corpus callosum, which passes information between the two halves. Still, we see people have tendencies to habitually use or be better at right or left brain functions. Many in the vision field feel that eye exercises can integrate and balance these brain functions.

One way to keep both sides of the brain engaged is by making sure that the brain is not suppressing (shutting off) vision in one eye. By seeing with both eyes, we send signals to both halves of our brain to process in their unique ways. There are ways to shut off the left brain function so dominant in our society, in order to allow the right brain its time. One way is through meditation. Another way is by patching the eye, covering the dominant eye (often the right) for about 20 minutes. (See Eye Patching).

Now let's go back to the eye-brain connection. Remember the cat in Sperry's experiments? The right brain processes in a spatial, holistic, artistic, emotional manner. The left brain is analytical, sequential, discrete and logical. What is not as well known is that each eye has its own unique personality, processing intake in one of these two ways. When you cover your right eye and look with your left eye, you are probably processing in a right-brained, holistic, spatial way. Conversely, when you are looking with your right eye, you are probably processing in a left-brained, logical, analytical manner.

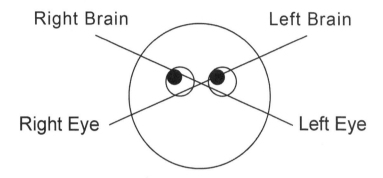

Several true stories will serve as examples of this. In the first instance, I was practicing patching, meaning putting a patch over one eye to strengthen the other eye's ability to see and to stay "engaged." I noticed that I immediately began having some disagreements with my husband. I was insistent that he empathize with me on some emotional issues, while he persisted in looking at them logically. It was as if we were speaking different languages or talking across a great chasm. We were at such great odds that we finally had to suspend our discussion. When I realized that I had been patching my right eye (left brain), in effect shutting off my logical, analytical faculties and processing everything emotionally, I understood why. Later, with "both my eyes wide open," we were able to come to agreement on the topic. On another occasion, he asked me a question about taxes, something that for me had a high emotional charge. Without thinking, I slapped my hand over my left eye (covering the right brain, emotional) and answered him quite logically. He was satisfied and I had no emotional reaction. While I do not recommend covering one eye to shut down that eye's brain function, I tell these stories to illustrate the truth and power of the eyes' relationship to brain function.

A quick test may be done to find out which of your eyes is more right-brained (emotional) and which is more left-brained (logical). Think of something highly emotional, where you can actually *feel* the emotion. As you continue to feel the emotion, cover your right eye. Notice if the emotions intensify or abate and what you think about. Then cover your left eye and notice how you feel and what you think. One eye will tend to be more emotional and the other more logical.

To experience using different brain functions, take a piece of paper and copy this picture:

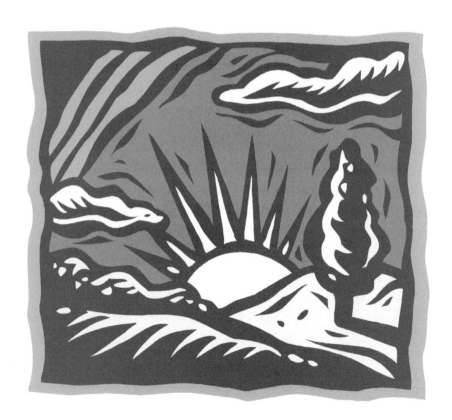

When you have finished, take another piece of paper, turn the picture upside down and copy it again.

The upside-down drawing is usually much more accurate because we don't have the influence of seeing a meaningful picture. We are just copying lines and shading. When we copied the right-side-up drawing, our symbolic processing was also engaged, which uses our language pathways, as the picture we were seeing had some meaning. Originally presented in *The New Drawing on the Right Side of the Brain* by Betty Edwards, this technique is incorporated today in many drawing classes.

Right and Left Brain Functions Related to Finger Push-Ups Exercise

Once the partner has pointed out the differences between the right and left eyes in their abilities to track the finger, it is an easy transition to talk about the person's logical, analytical abilities compared to their intuitive, emotional abilities. If a person's left eye has more trouble tracking, ask about the area with which they have trouble or where they have shut down their holistic, spatial, emotional and intuitive abilities. On the other hand, if a person's right eye seems less adept, ask them if they have difficulties in the logical, analytical areas of life. If a person's right eye is the stronger, find out if their logical, analytical abilities are more dominant. If their left eye is the stronger, ask them about their facility and interest in feelings, music, sports, intuition and creativity.

Workshop participants frequently relate stories about which brain function is predominant in their lives. One whose left eye is strong and right eye is less engaged may tend to process everything intuitively and emotionally and have trouble with dry, precise analytical functions. Another, whose right eye is strong and whose left eye seems "lazy," may relate a deep emotional wounding that has made them wary of delving very deeply into any emotional feelings. Neither function is better or worse, right or wrong. It is exciting to discover how the functioning of your own eyes reflects your characteristics and tendencies in right and left brain processing.

Once your partner has given you feedback on how your right and left eyes function in the Finger Push-Up exercise and you become aware of how your eyes are functioning, the next step is to get both eyes to work together equally. In this way you are also teaching both sides of your brain to stay engaged. You can increase the wholeness of your brain processing by insuring that both eyes function well and equally. This simple Finger Push-Up exercise can literally improve and balance your brain functioning!

The best way to take in information, make good decisions and relate successfully to others is to use both sides of the brain, both the holistic/emotional and the analytical/logical, at the same time. Either way by itself is partial and lopsided. Therefore, we are more balanced logically and emotionally when we see simultaneously and equally well with both eyes.

Palming—Exercise Completion

After doing this exercise for several minutes, feeling the stretch and beginning to sense the engagement of each eye as well as jumps and glitches, the exerciser should relax and rest the eyes. Rub your hands together to create a little friction and warmth. Then cup your palms gently over your closed eyes, completely blocking out the light and warming them (palming). Quietly take deep, slow breaths and relax your eyes.

Check Your Vision

Usually an improvement can be seen after doing the Finger Push-Up exercise, so this is another good time to re-check your vision. While standing or holding the paper the same distance away as before, notice how well you can see now. If there is an improvement, let that be your motivation to do these Eye Yoga exercises on a regular, daily basis! If you don't notice an improvement yet, relax and be patient. Allow your eyes time to improve.

Daily Eye Yoga Exercise

After initially doing this with a partner, you are ready to do this each day on your own. Use your own finger to get your eyes to move inward and back out together. Feel each one doing its part. If one has tended to be weaker or less engaged, cover the other eye and do the Push-Ups with the weaker eye to strengthen it. Then do it with both eyes to ensure their cooperation and coordination.

(Optional) Checking to See if Your Head is Straight

Do you habitually tilt your head to one side without being aware of it? One way to check this and correct it is to put your finger out six to twelve inches from your face and look past it to the distance to make your finger split into two images. If one is lower than the other, adjust your head tilt until the two images line up.

OTHER USES

Finger Push-Ups are very good for a far-sighted person, as they practice getting the eyes to converge at shorter distances. They are also good for presbyopia, or "short-arm" syndrome. This is when a person begins to lose the ability to see things up close like a restaurant menu, and their arm isn't long enough to hold it far enough away to see! If you find that you cannot see something up close, doing a few Finger Push-Ups to adjust your eyesight may help you see more clearly.

CHAPTER 6

V-IN AND V-OUT

This next exercise is a significant part of your Eye Yoga workout. Apart from merely exercising your eyes, there is "more than meets the eye" in this one. Most of our vision happens in the brain. It is the brain's interpretation of the signals from the eyes that creates vision. The brain can literally shut down vision in one or both eyes (called suppression), as well as increase or decrease visual clarity. Even when both eyes are seeing (not suppressed), each eye gives a different perspective, from a different place in space. This is essential for depth perception. In this exercise, your eyes are encouraged to work together to create a kind of "double vision." It cannot be done successfully if one eye isn't seeing, or if the brain has suppressed vision in one of your eyes.

In this exercise, you will be looking in front of (near point) or beyond (far point) your two fingers, which are held up in a V formation. While focusing on a near point, you will also be aware of your two fingers in the background, which will seem to split into two Vs. And when you are focusing on a far point, you will also be aware of your two fingers in the foreground, which will also seem to split into two Vs. Your eyes must work together to create a kind of "double vision." This is the "team teaching" exercise—getting both eyes to coordinate and work together, encouraging depth perception. Practicing this will also make the next exercises easier to do.

With that cryptic introduction, let's begin with what this exercise does. In addition to keeping both eyes engaged (not suppressing vision in one eye), it teaches the eyes to work together. By insuring that both eyes are seeing, it works on depth perception. It also develops flexibility, speed, depth perception, precision and a wider range of movement.

Some people find it easier to aim their eyes at a near point while others find it easier at a far point. We tend to use our eyes more for what is easier, which limits our full range of eye movement. This exercise works on both near point and far point, thus balancing the way we function. Basically, these are good, general exercises for everybody, since they engage the brain as well as the eye muscles.

PERSPECTIVE

As was explained above, each eye gives a different perspective. Let's first experience this difference in perspective. Look at an object in front of you (either near or far). A pencil works well for this. Have your partner hold a pencil in front of your face, several feet away. First, cover one eye, then the other, in fairly rapid succession. You will see the object shift back and forth, side to side. Each eye is looking at the object from a different place, so the object should appear to be jumping or changing position as you look with first one eye, then the other. This is a bit like two people who, no matter how similar, still have different outlooks.

Now, hold your two index fingers vertically, straight out in front of you, one, a foot or so from your nose, and the other at arm's length. While looking at the front finger nearest your nose, gently jiggle the back finger. Notice that the back finger appears double.

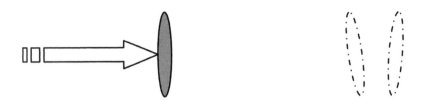

Now, look at the back finger and gently jiggle the front finger. Notice the front finger is now double.

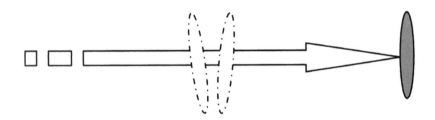

Why is this? Whatever you aim both eyes at, you see as a single object, and everything else is doubled. So as to not make you crazy, the brain phenomenally tunes out this confusion of seeing every-thing in the periphery as double. It is a marvel that our brains can actually change the two different pictures created by the two differ-ent viewpoints of our eyes into one picture. You can, however, if you pay close attention, see the slightly different pictures as you look at an object first with one eye then the other, or as you look back and forth between the near and far fingers.

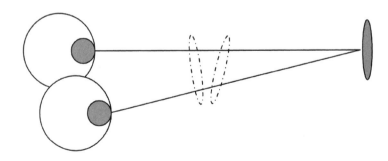

EQUIPMENT NEEDED

By holding your index and middle fingers in a V out in front of you, you have all the equipment needed. "Have fingers, will travel!" It's like carrying your gym equipment around with you so you can practice in spare moments. How about that for no excuses?

V-IN

Hold your two fingers (index and middle) out in front of you in a V shape with some space (one to two inches) in between them. Hold them at a comfortable distance from your nose in front of you (about 18 inches). Slightly cross your eyes so your eyes are focusing on a spot in front of the finger V until you see three fingers. Put your attention on the center one. Clearly see the tip where the two (imaginary) fingers come together.

THREE FINGERS:

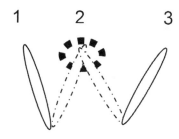

FOUR FINGERS:

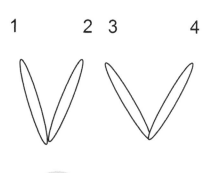

If you have trouble making three fingers, put a pen between the fingers and watch the pen as you slowly move it toward your nose. You may start to notice the two fingers splitting into three or four. If your eyes cross (converge) too much, they will make four fingers, so relax your eye-crossing a little. The idea of using a pen is to teach your eyes where to aim and focus, i.e., in front of your fingers. Once you have seen three fingers using the pen, try it without the pen by looking at the space where the pen had been.

Palming—Exercise Completion

Practice getting three fingers a number of times until you can do it easily. Then relax, cover your closed eyes with your cupped hands and palm for a few minutes, making sure to breathe easily and fully and to relax any tension in your eyes and body.

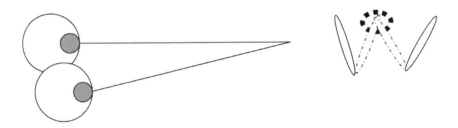

Partner's Job

While the V-In and V-Out exercises don't really require help from a partner, the partner may do some of the following to provide encouragement and support:

- It may be helpful to hold your two fingers out in front for the person so they can focus their attention on seeing three fingers.

- If the person cannot get three fingers, hold the pen in between the V shape formed by the fingers and slowly move the pen in toward their nose and out again toward the fingers. This gives the person something to focus on as they watch the fingers in the background.

- Remind them to relax and to breathe. Often people concentrate so much that they forget to breathe.

V—OUT

Again, hold your index and middle fingers out in front of you in a V shape, spreading the fingers so there is some space between them. Hold them the same comfortable distance from your nose in front of you. Look through and past your fingers to the distance until you see three fingers. You may have to adjust how far in the distance you look to make the three. You may also experiment with holding your fingers closer or farther away. Once you see the three fingers, put your attention on the center finger. Focus on it.

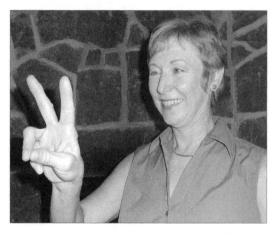

If you have trouble making three fingers this way, bring your fingers up close to your nose and look through them into the distance. Bring your fingers out slowly, continually looking afar, until you see three fingers.

Palming – Exercise Completion

Practice doing this a number of times, then relax by covering your closed eyes with your cupped hands and palm for a few minutes.

Now, with your fingers as your traveling companions, you can practice the V-In and V-Out exercises anywhere. It takes only a few minutes, so do them both frequently.

JUMP Vs—V-IN AND V-OUT

Once you have mastered the V-In and V-Out exercise, you are ready for the expert level. First do the V-In, then do the V-Out. You will move your eyes from looking up close for convergence to looking afar for divergence as you jump back and forth between the two. Anyone looking at your eyes would see them alternate from turned in to turned out.

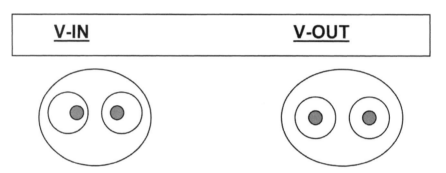

You may notice the middle finger being farther away in V-In and closer to you in the V-Out. This is one way to check to be sure you are actually doing both V-In and V-Out.

Eventually, you will be able to jump smoothly and quickly back and forth.

Jump Vs Instructions

- Holding your fingers in front of you at a comfortable distance, do a V-In by aiming the eyes at a near point in front of them, getting three fingers. Focus on the "middle finger," which may appear farther away than the other two.

- Now, shift the eyes to the distance beyond the finger V, doing a V-Out to get three fingers. Again focus on the "middle finger," which now should appear closer.

- Continue shifting between V-In and V-Out.

- Take breaks, as needed.

- Increase the speed with which you jump from one to the other.

- Be sure to palm afterward and release any tensions you may have in your eyes, shoulders and neck.

Other Variations

Next, try moving your fingers as you keep your focus on that middle finger. First get three fingers. Then slowly move your fingers toward and away from your face, in a trombone-like motion, only as quickly as you can keep seeing three fingers. Below are some movement variations to try:

In and out like a trombone	Right and left
Up and down	In diagonals
In circles	In Figure 8s

Troubleshooting

If you continue to see only two fingers, it is possible that you are only seeing with one eye. The brain can actually shut down or suppress vision in one eye without your even being aware of it. In such a case, you would not be able to see three fingers. To find out if you are suppressing, or only seeing with one eye, go to the Knots on a String exercise (page 73).

Below is a depiction of how you are able to see three fingers, by using both eyes:

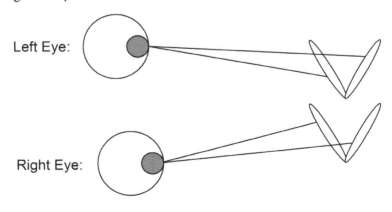

Left Eye:

Right Eye:

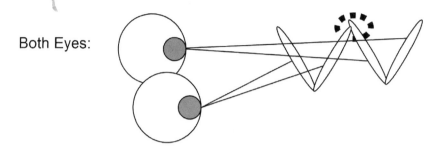

Both Eyes:

CHAPTER 7

SEE CIRCLE VARIATIONS

SEE IN – CONVERGENT SEE CIRCLES

The following is an additional exercise to practice eye convergence and to make sure both eyes are working together. Practicing this will make the next exercise, Knots on a String, easier as well. Hold the circles about a foot and a half from your face. Now cross your eyes slightly and look at the space in front of them.

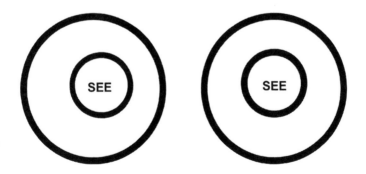

Get Three Circles

The object is to get your eyes to see three sets of circles instead of two. The third set should have the SEEs lined up on top of each other so they look like one. Focus on the middle SEE. Below is what you should be seeing. If the middle SEEs are not aligned, make sure your head is straight, not tilted to one side.

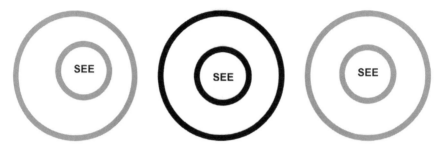

If you have trouble making three sets, put a pen in between the two circles on the paper. Focus on the pen and slowly move it toward your face. As you do this, be aware of the circles in the background by using your peripheral vision. You may notice the two sets of circles splitting into four, then moving back into three. If you see four sets, it means you have over-converged (crossed your eyes too much). If you are still having trouble getting and holding three circle sets, experiment with moving the pen slowly toward your nose and back out, while observing the circles in the background. Do this until you get three sets of circles. Eventually, when your eyes get the idea of where to aim, you will not need the pen to see the three circle sets. (The pen is a crutch to help direct your eyes to a point in front of the circles). When you can see three sets of circles, slowly remove the pen and continue to focus where the pen was. Note: If the middle SEEs are not aligned, make sure your head is straight and not tilted to one side. Sometimes it takes awhile to get the circles to line up. Then, all of a sudden, your brain will lock it in and you will clearly see three. If you lose them, take a slow, deep breath and try again. With practice it will become easy.

Make The Word "SEE" Clear

Once the three sets have "stabilized" and you can hold the over-lapped circles without losing them, focus on the middle word SEE. Can you make SEE clear? If not, ask your brain to "see clear." Some people may not be able to do this at first because they cannot yet clear words at this distance. With practice they will be able to see SEE clearly. In the meantime, imagine SEE clearly.

Find the Closer Circle

As you are looking at the middle circle set, notice which one of the circles is closer to you, the smaller or the larger. This may take a little time to see, but it will come. By seeing the SEE clearly and focusing on it, the two middle circle sets should begin to have a 3-D effect, with one circle closer and the other farther away. The SEE in the middle set of circles should look like it is inset deeper, farther away. The outer circle should look closer, as you are seeing 3-D. If you cannot see it at first, imagine that you are seeing it. It is fun when you can get the depth of the 3-D effect and the larger circle looks much closer to you.

Palming—Exercise Completion

Practice getting the three circle sets a number of times. Then relax by covering your closed eyes with your cupped hands and palm for a few minutes.

More Stretching Variations

- Look away from the circles, then look back to the circles and get three again. SEE the middle word clearly and notice the smaller circle appears farther away. Repeat several times. Then close and cover your eyes with cupped hands to relax them, as before.

- Get the three circles and hold them, focusing on the middle SEE, keeping it clear. Now slowly move the page in toward your nose. If you lose the three or SEE becomes unclear, begin again. Now, move the page away from your nose as far as you can. Maintain the three circles and keep SEE clear. Start over if you lose the three circles or SEE is unclear. When you can do this easily, move the page back and forth like a trombone, all the while focusing on the middle set of circles and their SEE. Finish by palming.

- Move the page in different patterns other than close and away, such as:

      Right and left
      Up and down
      In diagonals
      In circles
      In Figure 8s horizontally and vertically

Finish by palming.

SEE OUT — DIVERGENT SEE CIRCLES

Once you can get the above convergent circles, try diverging your eyes. In fact, if you had trouble with the convergent circles, doing these divergent circles may be easier for you. Look at the two sets of circles again. This time, look *beyond* them until you again see three sets.

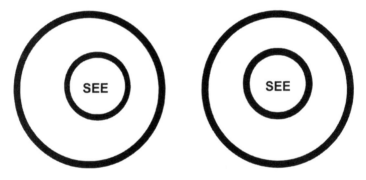

Focus on the SEE in the middle set as before until you can SEE it clearly. Once it is clear, find the closer circle. This time the inner circle should look closer and the outer circle farther away. That is how you can tell whether your eyes have converged or diverged.

If the small circle is farther away, your eyes are converging.

If the small circle is closer, your eyes are diverging.

Palming – Exercise Completion

Practice getting the three circle sets a number of times. Then relax by covering your closed eyes with your cupped hands and palm for a few minutes.

More Stretching Variations

- Look away from the circles, then look back to the circles and get three again. SEE the middle word clearly and notice the smaller circle appears closer. Repeat several times. Then close and cover your eyes with cupped hands to relax them, palming as before.

- Get the three circles and hold them, focusing on the middle SEE, keeping it clear. Now slowly move the page in toward your nose. If you lose the three or SEE becomes unclear, begin again. Now, move the page away from your nose as far as you can. Maintain the three circles and keep SEE clear. Start over if you lose the three circles or SEE is unclear. When you can do this easily, move the page back and forth like a trombone, all the while focusing on the middle set of circles and their SEE. Finish by palming.

- Move the page in different patterns other than close and away, such as:

Right and left
Up and down
In diagonals
In circles
In Figure 8s horizontally and vertically

Finish by palming.

CIRCLE JUMPS—ALTERNATING CONVERGENCE AND DIVERGENCE

To try the expert level, you will first look in front of the circles and converge your eyes, making the inner circle farther away. Then you will look beyond the circles and diverge your eyes to make the inner circle closer. You will be going from See In to See Out and back. Your eyes are moving in and then out, in and out, as they jump from In to Out. You may feel a stretch. Eventually, you will be able to jump smoothly and quickly, back and forth. Anyone watching your eyes will see your eyes move closer together and then farther apart.

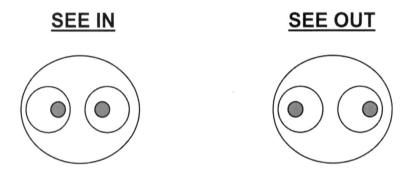

SEE IN   **SEE OUT**

Here are specific instructions for doing the Circle Jumps:

- Place the page at a comfortable distance from your nose. Aim the eyes at a near point in front of the paper and get three sets of circles. Focus on the word SEE clearly and notice the larger circle being closer.

- Now, shift the eyes to the distance beyond the paper and get three sets of circles as you look afar. Focus on the word SEE clearly and notice the smaller circle being closer.

- Continue shifting between near circles and far circles. Make sure SEE is clear before shifting again.

- Take breaks and palm, as needed.

- Increase the speed with which you shift your focus and make sure SEE is clear.

- End the exercise by palming for a few minutes.

The diagram below shows where your eyes are actually aiming when you See In (converge) and when you See Out (diverge):

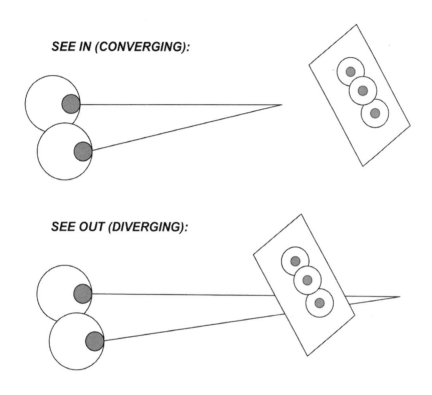

SEE IN (CONVERGING):

SEE OUT (DIVERGING):

NOTE

If this exercise is difficult and you cannot get or hold three circle sets, go back to the V-In and V-Out exercises. Sometimes they are easier to do, because you don't have the obstruction or distraction of the paper. In the V-Out exercise, you can look *through* your fingers to the distance without having the paper block your sight.

Head Tilt: You can tell if your head is straight or tilted to one side by whether the middle SEEs line up exactly. If one is higher, tilt your head slightly until they line up.

Farsighted people (those who see better far away than up close) can usually do the Circle Out exercise easier than the Circle In. Near-sighted people (those who see better close up than far away) usually find the Circle In exercise easier.

MAKING CLEAR CIRCLES
EQUIPMENT VARIATION

Doing this exercise can be much easier if you copy the two sets of SEE Circles onto a piece of clear plastic. Cut each set into a square, and use the two to practice this exercise. Having the circle sets on clear plastic makes the exercise easier to do because your eyes are not distracted by the paper. You can see through the clear plastic, allowing your eyes to converge and diverge with ease. This is particularly useful for SEE Out Circles, since when you use the paper, you can't see through it and have to imagine seeing afar. You can look at objects at different far distances until you successfully get three circle sets. It is easy to carry these little plastic squares with you in your wallet, so you can pull them out to practice any time. For example, if I had trouble reading something up close, I would actually pull these out, practice and improve my eyesight on the spot.

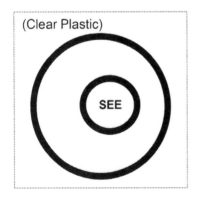
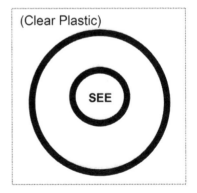

CHAPTER 8

KNOTS ON A STRING

The string exercise builds on what you practiced in V-In, V-Out and in SEE Circles.

- **Focus**: In terms of Eye Yoga, you are practicing changing your focus at different distances, much like the lens of a camera does when changing focus from portrait to panoramic. It is important for the eyes to shift smoothly and effortlessly from one focus point to another.

- **Aiming Flexibility:** When we look at a distance, our eyes are in the middle position. When we look at something close up, our eyes turn in or slightly cross.

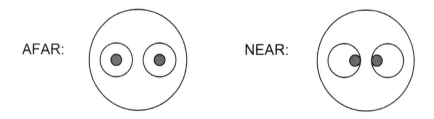

AFAR: NEAR:

- **Aiming Precision:** You are also getting feedback in this exercise about whether you are really aiming your eyes at a specific place in space or whether you just think you are.

- **Teaming:** This exercise also lets you know if you are using both eyes together without partially or wholly shutting down your vision in one of your eyes (called suppression). It gives feedback on how well your brain is processing the information from your eyes. You can actually tell your brain to turn on or off the sight in one eye! This helps you learn to control your brain-eye partnering to activate more of its potential, both in seeing and in thinking.

PREPARATION

Remember the finger focus perspective experiment at the beginning of V-In and V-Out, where you focused on a finger in front or behind? When you aimed your eyes at the finger in front, the back finger doubled, and vice versa.

In V-In, V-Out, you aimed your eyes at the space in front of or beyond the fingers to make the objects seem to double.

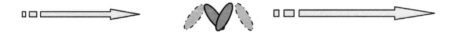

In Knots on a String, you will be focusing on a knot along the string, which in effect makes it single, while the rest of the string looks double, like an X through the knot.

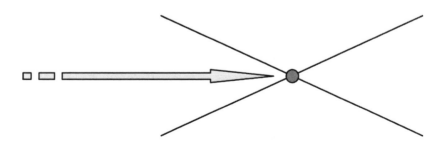

As we've said before, each eye has a slightly different vantage point, so the string will look different for each eye.

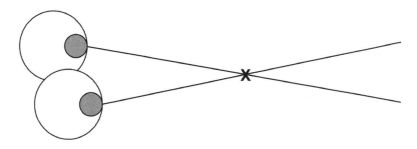

If you are only looking with one eye, you will only see one string.

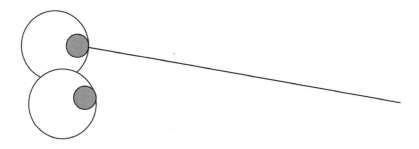

If your focus point is not on the knot itself, you may see two knots.

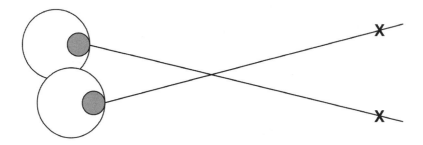

HOW TO DO THE KNOTS
ON A STRING EXERCISE

For this exercise you will need a string 4–6 feet long. Put knots in it every foot or so.

CAUTION: This exercise can be stressful or tiring. Just as with any exercise regimen, begin slowly and monitor yourself. Take breaks by looking far in the distance and/or cupping your hands over your closed eyes.

With a Partner

Start with a few deep, relaxing breaths. Have the partner hold one end of the string, standing about 4–6 feet out in front of you. You take the other end of the string and hold it up to the end of your nose or just under it. Make sure you are sitting or standing up straight and tall, relaxing the rest of your body.

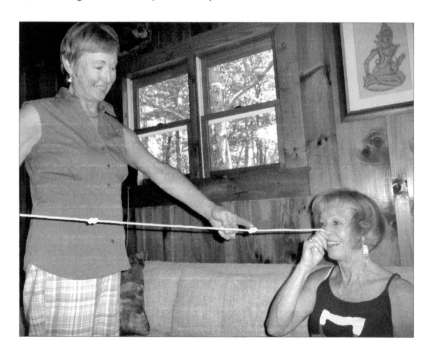

Your partner should then point to one of the knots, maybe 2–3 feet in front of your nose, for you to focus on. Check to be sure that you can comfortably bring the knot into focus, meaning that it is not too close or far away for you to see with ease.

As you look at the knot, do you see two strings going into it? And do you see two strings leading away from the knot? As explained above, if both eyes are looking at the knot, you will see two strings, one trajectory for each eye. Because our brain can merge double visions, it may take some attention before you become aware of the two strings. Breathe, relax, and notice what you see.

Partner's Job

The partner's job in this exercise is to hold the string fairly taut, using just enough tension so it is straight; to direct the person's focus to a knot; and to watch their eyes. Ask the person if they can see two strings going into the knot; and two leaving the other side. If they can do this, have them focus on different knots along the string to check to see if at each position they still see the string X through the knot. Your job is also to watch the person's eyes to see if both eyes are engaged and looking at the knot. If one eye is turned in and the other is sort of staring out into space, the probability is that the person will not be seeing two strings or will be seeing the strings form some other pattern.

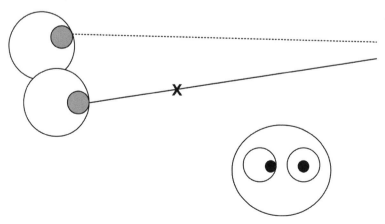

Work with the person to get them to successfully focus on the knot with both eyes, so that they see two strings forming an X with the knot in the center. Sometimes this is just a question of the eyes understanding what is wanted. It may take a moment for the person to become aware of the two strings. Occasionally, the person may think they are focusing on the knot when in fact they are only seeing it in their peripheral vision. Their actual focus is elsewhere.

What to Do if the Person Cannot See Two Strings Forming an X

In the Eye Yoga workshops, roughly 25% of the participants cannot see the string X at first. In these cases, assuming there is no physical reason such as blindness in one eye, it is quite possible that their brain is shutting down or suppressing vision in one eye. Your job will be to get your partner to see with both eyes. Here are some suggestions for the partner to try:

1. Ask the person to tell both of their eyes to work together to engage and see. Sometimes this works, as the person's brain is able to communicate to their eyes.

2. Put your fingers at the knot to help the person better focus their attention on it.

3. If these do not work, your next step will be to find out which eye is "not seeing."

First, you need to understand what each eye is seeing. The right eye sees the string coming from the left side of the head, whereas the left eye sees the string coming from the right.

A. RIGHT EYE: B. LEFT EYE:

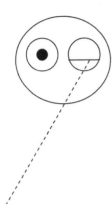   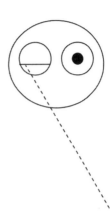

There are two ways to find out which eye is seeing. One is to ask the person to explain which direction the string is going, as in the drawings above. The other is to cover first one eye and then the other with your hand or a piece of paper to find out which eye is seeing. If the person is seeing with the right eye, as in position A above, and you cover that right eye, the string will "jump" to the position in B above, as they change to seeing it with their left eye.

Once you know which eye has shut down, you can have the person concentrate on seeing with that eye. They may be able to talk to that eye, as in earlier exercises, encouraging it to do what they want. You may also practice having that eye see by covering the dominant eye, forcing the non-seeing eye to see the string, then removing your hand to encourage both eyes to see together. Do this a number of times, covering and uncovering the recalcitrant eye. This may take awhile, so don't lose patience. Eventually, the brain will get the idea, and suddenly the person will exclaim that they now see two strings! It may go back and forth between two and one for a while, as the person teaches both of their eyes to see together.

The really amazing thing that blows people's socks off is that one can actually tell their brain to turn on the sight in the eye that wasn't seeing! In Eye Yoga Workshops, I usually find a person who only sees one string to be the demo for the class. Say, for instance, that the person is only seeing the string with their right eye. I tell them to literally instruct their left eye to also see. I get them to have their brain instruct their left eye to see. When that happens and they exclaim that they can now see two strings, the class is amazed. They immediately want to try it for themselves.

Often the person can then instruct their left eye to shut down again, returning to one string, and then back on again for two strings. This ability of the brain to literally turn on or shut off vision can change one's whole paradigm for eyesight. Up until now, it has just been a few yoga stretches to exercise the eyes. By having an experience of literally turning on and off your vision, just imagine the many other possibilities!

I first learned this from Dr. Jacob Liberman in his book, *Light: Medicine of the Future.* He commented that he could see better than he was measured optometrically as seeing by instructing his eyes to see. When I was working to improve my distance sight, I tried this. I would tell my eyes to *focus* and to read a sign in the distance. Sure enough, for a split instance, the sign would be clear. Then it would return to fuzzy. Over time, I developed the ability to sharpen my eyesight when desired or needed. I could extend those "split instances" of clear sight to longer periods. I realized that I like my world a little fuzzy. I prefer to see things with soft edges and not so sharply delineated. It is prettier, somehow. So most of the time, when I don't need to see things with sharpness, I allow my body to envision the world in the way it is most comfortable. However, I have developed enough rapport with my eyesight that I can instruct my eyes to focus and to look sharp, to get the details that I need to see. And my eyes will obey. I listen to them and they listen to me.

I CAN SEE CLEARLY NOW: "I grew up in Toronto in a family of dedicated bowlers. These were 5-pin leagues, where the pins and balls are smaller than the familiar 10-pin game. By age ten, I wore glasses but still didn't see the pins clearly. One day, through intuition, I decided to really focus my attention on the distant pins before I threw the ball. Within seconds, I had a sudden flash of clarity where, by my intense desire and concentration, the pins appeared larger and closer. I felt the thrill of discovery.

"Each time I focused, the room seemed to consist of just myself and the lane leading to the pins. After bowling, my eyes stayed focused for longer periods of time. The muscles felt stronger. I threw strikes with increasing regularity and qualified for an adult tournament when I was a teen. Using this technique, I won a top prize. I practiced this and other eye exercises to train and improve my sight for outdoor sports like golf, baseball and Frisbee. While reading the manuscript of *Eye Yoga*, I recalled this exercise and now include it daily with increasing clarity, especially for reading without glasses. Thanks for your countless insights to improve our eyesight."

— Lance D. Ware, M.A., CHT

Another variation is to have the person who sees two X-ed strings get their brain to shut down vision in one eye so they only see one string. Sometimes the brain suppresses vision in one eye under stressful conditions. Have the person think of something with a very high emotional charge, really getting into the emotion. As they think of it, look at the knot on the string. It may cause them to shut down vision in one eye. It may be their left eye (right brain), which would then shut out the intensity of the emotion. Or if they feel the intense need to process emotionally, they may shut down their logical side (right eye, left brain). You may also have the person think about doing some onerous, distasteful intellectual task for them, like doing math or doing their taxes. You may ask them to add large numbers, like 394 and 268, in their head. This is another way to induce one string to disappear. Anything that stresses the person in either an emotional or analytical way may cause their brain to shut down the vision in one eye, reducing the vision to one string. Always end by having the person see two strings.

Palming – Exercise Completion

Once the person has successfully seen both strings making an X through the knot, they should relax their eyes by palming. Instruct the person to rub their hands together to create a little friction and warmth. Then have them cup their palms gently over their eyes, warming them and blocking out all the light. Have them quietly take deep, slow breaths and relax their eyes.

EYE-BRAIN CONNECTION

Once again, this exercise gives an insight into how your brain is functioning. Under stress (e.g., thinking of a highly emotional situation, the need to "perform" or even the need to see two strings), the brain may resort to looking at the situation in a habitually comfortable way by processing predominantly in a right-brained or a left-brained way. Your brain has the ability to shut down vision in your right eye if it wants to process emotionally, in a right-brained way, and it can shut out the vision in the left eye to process in a logical, left-brained way. Most people would never be aware that their brains have done this.

Robert Ornstein and David Galin (Ornstein, p. 33) conducted research on the brain's electrical activity in each hemisphere while subjects performed verbal and spatial activities. They found one side to be active while the other side "idled." Their opinion was that in most ordinary activities we alternate between the two modes, selecting one while inhibiting the other. Even though we need both modes, our brain, under stress, can shut off input temporarily from one eye in order to "control" which hemisphere is dominant.

"Why," you may ask, "should I even care whether I am seeing with one eye or with both?" Seeing with both eyes is a more balanced way of processing information and responding intelligently by engaging both sides of your brain. An overly logical, analytical person or an overly emotional person are both out of balance, not using all their faculties. It produces a lopsided way of responding and interacting. The brain may get into the habit of over-dependence on one way to the detriment of the whole. Like favoring one leg over another because it is weaker only worsens the discrepancy, encouraging our brain to keep both sides available is preferred.

In addition, seeing out of only one eye causes a person's vision to be two-dimensional instead of three-dimensional. The ability to have depth perception (3-D) is critical for such professionals as athletes and airline pilots. The world has such beauty when seen with depth!

Personal Experience: "One day, after working diligently for weeks on not suppressing, I looked out at a landscape and "saw" space for the first time! The whole world looked incredibly, emotionally beautiful! Seeing such space and depth between things was new and different. I sat for a long time just drinking in and appreciating that beauty, as I enjoyed seeing in 3-D. Even today, I can enjoy seeing the spaces between things as a little meditative respite."

— Jane Battenberg

The Knots on a String exercise will reveal how a person's brain is processing, if they see only one string at first. This information is usually kept unconsciously; the person isn't aware of how they tend to process. By relating the seeing pattern to the person's natural abilities and to what is going on in their life, the brain's suppression of sight in one eye may begin to make sense. For example, a person who sees only one string with their right eye (left brain) may be having some emotionally troubling events in their life. It could be a natural protection mechanism that the person uses to emotionally shut down by not seeing with their left eye (right brain). Maybe another person doesn't trust analytical people and needs to check out every situation intuitively and emotionally to tell to what degree they can trust it. The exercise shows whether a person is suppressing sight in one of their eyes. Whether it occurs only in stressful or particular situations or whether it is done constantly, it is important to actually experience the suppression. This builds on the previous exercises in showing the eyes' connection to right- and left-brain processing.

The second thing that this exercise teaches is that we can literally have our brain talk to the eyes and get them to see better. We can instruct our eyes to turn our sight on or off. If we can do that, we can also tell our eyes to sharpen the focus to see better close up or far away. Just knowing this fact can begin a rapport-building relationship between brain and eyes. It is at the core of this book's premise that there is an interlinking, integral relationship between the brain and our sight. How we see is how we think, and how we think is how we see.

BACK TO EYE YOGA

Daily Eye Yoga Exercise

After initially doing this with a partner, you are ready to do this each day on your own. You will need the knotted string. Even if you have trouble seeing a string X, this is a good exercise to practice.

- Attach one end of the knotted string to the wall, window, back of a chair or doorknob so it is just below eye level and there is nothing distracting the view.

- Hold the other end up to or just under your nose. (Keep good posture, not leaning over or jutting the head forward to meet the string).

- Focus on one knot at a time, ensuring that you see two strings forming an X with the knot in the middle. Practice with knots at all the different distances.

You can vary how you do this exercise depending on what you want to improve in your vision:

For Farsightedness and Presbyopia

- Begin at the far end of the string where it attaches to the wall. See the last knot clearly. You should see two strings going to a /\ as they point into the knot, if you are seeing with both eyes.

- Next, move your eyes toward your nose, focusing on one knot at a time. This time you should see a single X with the knot in the middle.

- Continue moving toward your nose, one knot at a time, getting an X through the middle of each knot as you go.

- Finish by aiming at your nose (or as close to it as you can) and seeing the string make a V from the knot to the wall.

For Nearsightedness and Myopia

- Begin by looking at your nose. You should see the string make a V from your nose to the wall.

- Now move your eyes away from your nose to the first knot. See a single knot and an X going through it.

- Continue moving one knot at a time toward the wall, seeing a single knot with an X through it.

- Finish with the /\ at the wall.

WHAT IF...

You Only See One String

The ability to see two strings is dependent on both eyes having a perspective, each one being slightly different, which makes the string look like an X. If you do not see two strings, your brain may be suppressing or shutting off vision in one eye. Suppression occurs periodically during the day in the average person, depending on their needs, fatigue and stress levels and what is going on situationally. Since suppression takes effort and energy (and over time could drive a person to some deeper form of adaptation), reducing suppression will bring a more efficient, binocular way of seeing.

If you only see one string, your brain is shutting off (suppressing) vision in one eye.

- Find out which eye isn't seeing:
  Left eye sees string going from right at near to left at far
  Right eye sees string going from left at near to right at far

- Blink each eye to see which string is being seen.

- Then, *tell* your eyes to see both strings.

You Don't Have an X

Instead of seeing an X, you might see one of these patterns:

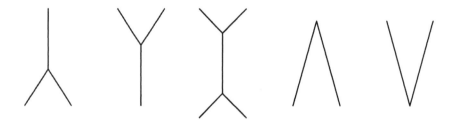

Even though you are seeing two strings, your eyes are still not seeing fully. To encourage your eyes to work together better and to see the string's full length, here are some suggestions.

- Blink one eye and then the other. Notice how the image changes. See if you can get your eye to restore the image to an X.

- If part of the X is missing, close one eye and then the other. This should restore the missing part of the string. Tell your mind to hold onto all parts longer and longer until they all stay there all the time. Just tell your mind to turn on and to see the full X. Encourage it to see it all.

- Use your imagination to fill in the blank. Look at another knot with an X through it. Remember this image as you look back to the knot where there wasn't an X yet. Continue shifting back and forth until you get the X.

- Tap one or both temples with your fingers to activate the brain to turn on all the way. You can also snap your finger(s) near your ear(s) or have someone do it for you to get the brain's attention.

- Tap the knot with your finger or a pointer to activate your eyes to see where the knot is, to get a fix on where it is in space. The touching and the movement help the eyes to fix attention on the knot.

The X is in Front of the Knot or Behind It

- Use your mind to "walk the X" into the knot.

- Encourage the X into the knot by putting a finger, pen or stick in the center of the X and moving it into the knot.

- Tap the knot between your fingers with a pen or a stick. Make it come alive in space.

- Visualize the X in the middle of the knot. Use the power of your imagination.

- Move the X further away from the knot then back toward it. Continue rocking it back and forth until you have control to move it into the knot.

- Aim your focus to the other side of the knot from the X and see where the X repositions itself. (If you see the X in front of the knot, look at the string just beyond the knot. Conversely, if the X is behind the knot, focus on the string just in front of the knot). Keep adjusting where you aim your eyes on the string until you get the X in the middle of the knot. Keep the X there as you then move your eyes' aim back into the knot.

If You See a Straight Line (| , \ or /)

If you do not see two strings, that means one eye is not seeing. Your eyes are not working together as a team and your brain has suppressed the image from one eye. You need to turn on the images from both eyes to get them coordinated.

- Tell your eyes to work together and stay turned on.

- Tap your temple(s).

- Snap your fingers near your ear(s).

- Visualize an X with eyes closed, then open your eyes and imagine seeing an X.

TALK TO YOUR BRAIN BECAUSE YOUR EYES ARE LISTENING

When you are seeing with both eyes, you can look out on a landscape and literally see the space between the objects, as if you could fall through that space if it were vertical, rather than horizontal. When you are seeing with only one eye, the landscape has more of a postcard, flat look. To test this, close one eye and look at the landscape. Now open both eyes and notice the difference. If you can see the spaces between things and depth in the landscape, you are seeing with both eyes and you are not shutting off vision in one eye. If, on the other hand, you see no difference, it could be that you are suppressing (not seeing with both eyes).

Once you get your brain to turn the double image back on, you can experiment with this brain control. Tell your brain to see just one string. Then tell it to see two strings again. Go back and forth from one string to two. Telling your brain to see that way starts a whole new relationship between you, your brain and your vision!

If you see the X all the time in this exercise, try turning two strings into one by getting your brain to suppress.

Experience Making Two Strings Turn to One

Each of the two strings that form the X relates to the functions of one hemisphere of the brain. If you see one string going / from left to right, it means you are seeing it with your right eye. It also means that you have probably shut off your left eye/right brain, the emotional-global part, and are processing in a left-brained, analytical, logical way. Conversely, if you see one string going \, from right to left, you are seeing with your left eye and have probably shut off your right eye/left brain. You have shut down most of your logical-analytical function.

If you see two strings forming an X through the knot, you can experiment to see if you can stress your brain enough to turn off the vision in one eye. There are several ways to do this:

- Think of something mentally challenging, like working a difficult math problem (such as 36 times 468) in your head. Or think of doing your taxes.

- Think of something emotionally charged; something that, as you think of it, still evokes strong emotional reactions.

- Tell your brain to turn off sight in one eye.

The purpose of turning off sight in one eye is to experience consciously what your brain probably does all the time outside of your awareness. Once you can experience your brain suppressing, you can tell it to turn the eye back on. Then in future circumstances, you will have more conscious control over your vision. You will develop a rapport between brain and eyes that allows them to respond to your desire to see well.

Most of us are unaware that our brain can shut down partial vision, of one whole eye or even of the near or distant part of an eye. Called "suppression," it happens more than we are aware. It can cause the 3-D effect to disappear and make blind spots in our vision. You can see how important it would be for pilots and athletes to practice non-suppression!

Have you ever noticed people turning their heads to one side as they talk to you, as if to emphasize looking with one eye? This is particularly noticeable when they are excited or emphatic. They are unconsciously "leading" with one brain hemisphere function.

Looking at you with the:

Right Eye   (Left Brain)—Logical-analytical
Left Eye   (Right Brain)—Emotional-global

Notice whether you turn your head to one side as you talk or listen. Do you ever close one eye or ever cover one eye as you talk? Be aware of what brain function your unconscious mind is emphasizing.

The brain can emphasize one side of the brain another way, by suppressing eyesight in one eye. You normally would not even be aware that it was doing this.

CHAPTER 9

PALMING/SUNNING

Now that you are winding down your Eye Yoga workout, it is time to move to the more relaxing exercises. As with your body muscles, it is important to teach your eye muscles to relax. Exercise expert Pete Cisco makes the point that strengthening your muscles occurs not during the workout itself but always happens in the rest or recovery period after the exertion. Since many vision problems are brought on by stress, this cool-down relaxation is very important.

Astigmatism—It is caused by the eye muscles pulling unevenly on the cornea. A warped or wrinkled cornea changes your focus, like looking through a wavy piece of glass.

Nearsightedness/Myopia—It can be brought on by mental/emotional stresses, frequently around starting school or puberty. It can also come from doing a lot of near-vision work, like reading, computer work, or needlepoint. When the eyes are kept at one distance for too long without a break (like repetitive motion strains), they fixate on that distance and lose flexibility.

Farsightedness and Presbyopia—When eyes aren't used very much for close-up work, they can lose the ability to adjust to it. When one uses glasses for close-up work, the glasses do the adjusting for the eyes, potentially making the eyesight worse. Fuzzy near vision can be brought on by not wanting to see things too closely (emotional, fearful, frustrated by too much detail).

It is recommended that you do palming, Sunning and a combination of both of them. Palming is the most important, so at least make sure to do this. We have recommended doing palming for a minute or so at the end of each exercise set. Now that you are at the end of the entire workout, you can relax for a longer time to give the eyes a deeper relaxation. Here is a brief overview of the three exercises:

Palming is good for relaxation of the eyes, the optic nerve, the face and the whole nervous system.

Sunning (eyes closed) is good for relaxation and reducing light-sensitivity. It bathes the inside of the eyeball with the rich nutrients of light, nourishing it as well as stimulating and waking up the inside of the eyeball—the rods, cones, everything.

Palming/Sunning Combo has added value. In addition to the benefits of each of these done separately, the combo of palming then Sunning stimulates the iris to open and close. This is very important to avoid or relieve light sensitivity.

PALMING

Palming is a way to relax your eyes, optic nerves, and the whole nervous system, which is also found in Rotté's holistic eyesight healing (p. 40). You shut out all the light to your eyes by cupping your palms over your closed eyelids. Even when you close your eyes, any external light goes through your eyelids, stimulating the retina and the optic nerve and then is passed on to the brain. Seeing is a function of the nervous system. Therefore, to give the whole vision-brain system a rest, we need complete darkness. Palming is a simple way to shut out the light for a full rest, and the good news is that you can never overdo it. The long-term, cumulative and more permanent effects of palming are usually measured in weeks or months, as they are short-lived at first.

> "Palming is one of the most effective methods of obtaining relaxation of all the sensory nerves."
>
> —William Horatio Bates, *Better Eyesight without Glasses*, p. 71

Partner's Job

The partner's job in this exercise is to read the following instructions to the person. Help create a calm, relaxed atmosphere for this. Watch the person for any unconscious tension and remind them to breathe and relax.

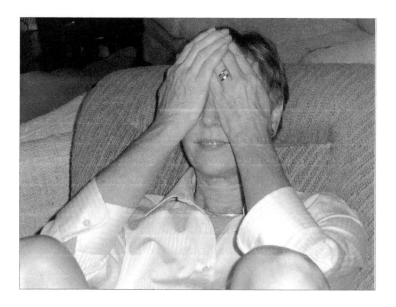

How to Palm

- Sit comfortably. Rest your elbows on a table or on your knees in a position that is relaxing. Some people prefer to lie on their back with elbows on their chest. Cover your closed eyes with your cupped hands, the heels of your hands on the occipital bone below your eyes and your fingers on your forehead. Rest your palms lightly so as not to touch your eyeballs. Adjust your hands to shut out all light.

- Feel your body's contact with the chair, your feet on the floor and your fingers on the forehead. Take full, easy and relaxed breaths, and be aware of any tension in your body. Just relax and let it go.

- Notice if you see colors, light flashes or patterns. These will eventually go away as the nervous system calms down and the optic nerve stops firing. Just notice what is there, be patient and continue to take in full, easy breaths. Sometimes it is helpful to remember something very black that you have seen in the past, like a black velvet dress, a jet black cat or being in a pitch black cave.

- If your body becomes uncomfortable, adjust it. If your mind wanders, bring it back to peacefulness. Endeavor to relax your mind as well as your eyes.

- Palm for as little as one minute, but as long as you wish, so long as it is restful to you.

- When you are ready to come out of palming, it is fun to sit back or just lie there and, with your eyes still closed, let your hands relax in your lap. Notice how much light actually comes through your eyelids. Enjoy the calm, sunny feeling and notice the peaceful relaxation you feel in your eyes and whole body.

- When you are ready to open your eyes, let them flutter open like soft butterfly wings. Let the light and the visual world come to you gently. Look around softly as you passively let the light touch you with its images. Enjoy a new way of seeing gently. Now see how long you can maintain this soft way of seeing as you re-engage with the world.

"When the mind is at rest nothing can tire the eyes, and when the mind is under a strain nothing can rest them."

– William Horatio Bates, *Better Eyesight without Glasses*, p. 41

SUNNING

"Truly the light is sweet, and a pleasant thing it is for the eyes to behold the sun."

—The Bible, Ecclesiastes 11:7

Sunning is a way to bathe your whole eyeball in light, by closing your eyes and letting the light come through your eyelids. Light is a nutrient. It is necessary for good eye health. We habitually use our eyes in limited patterns which doesn't let light in to all areas of the eyeball. Sunning is a way to bathe the whole eyeball in light. Like lying in the sun at the beach, Sunning your eyes relaxes them and releases accumulated eye tensions.

Sunning was first developed by Bates as a vision improvement technique. More than that, it stimulates our biological clocks, regulated by light (sunlight) and darkness. Our body is a living photoelectric cell, regulated by the sun's light energy. When we are deprived of sunlight, it has the same effect as jet lag.

Partner's Job

The partner's job in this exercise is to read the following instructions aloud to the person. Help create a calm, relaxed atmosphere for this. Watch the person for any unconscious tension. Also, remind them to breathe and relax.

How to Do the Sunning Technique

- Stand in front of a light source, preferably the sun. Gently close your eyes. Breathe in and out fully and easily in a regular rhythm.

- Move your head in an arc, starting with your nose pointing at one shoulder. Raise your nose up high, turning your head to point your nose down to the other shoulder. Let your eyes follow your nose as if looking straight ahead. Do this slowly and gently without excessive stretching or strain. Adjust the arc so it is comfortable for you.

- Notice the colors you see on the insides of your eyes. You may see warm colors, sparkles, after-images of the sun or mottled patterns. As you move your head to the side, notice how the bright and dark patterns shift.

- Feel the warmth of the light as it loosens and relaxes the eyeballs, eye muscles and any facial tension.

- Imagine you are a stick of butter put out in the sun and feel yourself softening and melting. Now let your thoughts melt away just like the butter and allow your mind to relax as well.

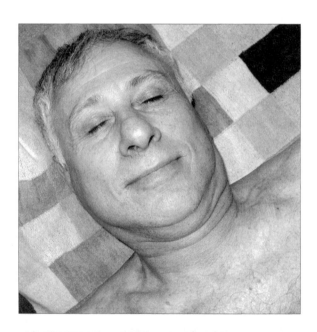

Sunning is done with the eyes closed.

Flicker Variation

A variation is to let the outstretched fingers of each hand cross over each other to create a flicker on your closed eyelids, like a strobe light. This stimulates the pupils as well as the brain. Because the brain pays attention to differences rather than that which is the same, the flickering wakes up your brain.

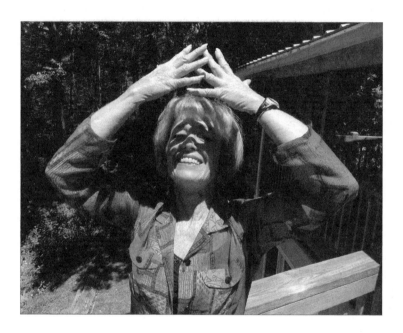

PALMING/SUNNING COMBO

Many people have light sensitivity, where they need dark sunglasses in full sun, and bright light hurts their eyes. This exercise stimulates the pupils to open and close quickly and completely in response to changes in light intensity. By exercising the pupils to open and close, you can improve your eyes' ability to react to bright or dim light. When a person uses sunglasses, there is no need for their pupils to keep this level of proficiency. The sunglasses actually keep the pupil from making the Eye Yoga movements needed to reduce sensitivity. Palming/Sunning can balance out the weakening effects of sunglasses.

The combination of palming and Sunning alternates between washing the eyeballs with filtered light and bathing them in darkness. This alternation stimulates the pupil to close and open as it adjusts from dark to light and back again. This alternation is a workout for the muscles, both for range and speed of the open/close motion. "Use it or lose it," as they say.

Partner's Job

The partner's job in this exercise is to read the following instructions to the person. Help create a calm, relaxed atmosphere for this. Watch the person for any unconscious tension and remind them to breathe and relax.

How to Do the Palming/Sunning Combo

- Face the sun (or other light source) and begin Sunning in a smooth, relaxed way **_with your eyes closed_**. Do this for a few minutes.

- Next, cover your eyes with the palms of your hands. Remember to maintain your full, easy breathing. Do the palming for the same amount of time as the Sunning technique or longer. Sometimes it is nice to turn away from the sun to get more darkness.

- Turn back to the sun for more sunbathing, then away and palm for the soothing darkness.

- Repeat for as long as you wish and enjoy the relaxed, alert and refreshed feeling this brings to your eyes and your whole nervous system.

"When the sun is shining I can do anything; no mountain is too high, no trouble too difficult to overcome."

— Wilma Rudolph, first American runner to win three gold medals in the same Olympic Games (Rome, 1960)

CHAPTER 10

FINISHING UP

PATCHING

This exercise does not need a partner. It is an optional exercise for your daily Eye Yoga workout. It is used to independently strengthen both eyes and both sides of the brain. Frequently, one eye will work harder or be more dominant than the other. It is important to have each of your eyes exercise independently, just as in a gym you exercise each leg independently, and then both legs together, to bring both to the same strength and stamina. Independent strength is an important prerequisite to having both eyes work together as a team.

EYE-BRAIN CONNECTION

One way to keep both sides of the brain engaged is by making sure that the brain is not suppressing (shutting off) vision in one eye. By seeing with both eyes, we send signals to both halves of our brain to process in their unique ways. There are ways to shut off the left brain function, so dominant in our society, to allow the right brain its time. One such way is through meditation. Another way is by eye patching.

Patching an eye allows the uncovered eye its own experience of performing the visual tasks required of it. It can experience its strengths and weaknesses, its unique personality and its own identity. This takes into account that each eye processes information in a different manner. As we have said earlier, the eye usually processes according to its opposite brain hemisphere. The right eye may process mostly in a left-brained way, whereas the left eye may process mostly in a right-brained way.

RIGHT EYE	Left-Brained Processing	Logical, Sequential, Analytical, Yang
LEFT EYE	Right-Brained Processing	Wholistic, Artistic, Global, Emotional, Yin

Strengthening each eye is actually, in a sense, strengthening each brain function. You operate better in the world, make better decisions, relate to people better, and generally are smarter when you have both sides of your brain operating together. Just as you see three-dimensional depth when both eyes are functioning together, you also process information multi-dimensionally with left and right brain functions working together in partnership. Shutting down vision in one of your eyes is, in effect, shutting off a large part of visual input to one of your brain hemispheres. Patching allows you to strengthen each eye/brain input so that when you see with both eyes, each will be doing its part rather than a weaker one relying on the other eye to pull the weight, so to speak.

HOW TO PATCH

When patching, it is important to be in a safe environment that fosters exploration and experimentation. This means that you should not patch when you are driving or when you are expected to be functioning fully, such as at work. Suggested times are at home or when you are in a relaxed environment.

Buy an eye patch (usually found in drug stores) that fits so the covered eye will still be open while remaining in the dark. Or you can take two old, inexpensive pairs of sunglasses. Pop the right lens out of one and the left lens out of the other. Use opaque tape, such as electrician's or duct tape, or tape black paper over the remaining lenses. Using the glasses instead of an eye patch allows for some peripheral vision and light to come to the patched eye, so it does not just shut down and stop functioning. Either method of patching will work.

Patch one eye for up to 20 minutes at a time. Start with 5–10 minutes and work up. Then patch the other eye. You may want to keep a journal or make some notes about what you experience with each eye patched.

As you patch, notice what is different from seeing with both eyes together. Sometimes the world will look brighter or darker with one eye. Make note of any emotions that come up. Walk around and take in the environment. Experiment with different activities such as reading, personal conversations, doing complex calculations or banking, sitting quietly, listening to music, preparing dinner, walking outside in nature, doing creative arts, crafts or writing. Notice any body sensations, emotions, or mind chatter/thoughts that are there. Many people find their right eye to be more left-brained, yang, logical and detailed, and the left eye to be more right-brained, yin, emotional, intuitive and global. Experiment with your own eyes to see what is true for you.

Partner Exercises

Although it is not necessary to practice this with a partner, here are some fun things you can do together to explore patching.

- While patching, go outside, take a walk or hike in a park or the woods, or go to a playground.

- Talk to each other about various subjects while you are in close proximity, having the patcher notice shifts and nuances in this experience. Experiment with different distances to see if this makes any difference in thoughts and emotions.

- Have your partner ask you to perform different math problems in your head, such as large additions or divisions. Notice your reactions: whether it is easy, difficult or frustrating. What differences do you notice between the two eyes?

- Choose a topic that has some emotional charge: a fearful situation, a person who makes you angry or politics, for example. Talk about this with your partner and notice how you feel. Then switch the patch to the other eye and notice any differences in thoughts and emotions.

Stories

"When I first patched my dominant right eye, I found I became very timid and afraid. Normally I am very athletic; however, when my sister and I went for a walk in the woods during one of these patching periods, I had to hold onto her arm as I fearfully, cautiously made my way along the path."

"I found I could relate much better to my husband when I covered my left eye (right brain, emotional), which meant I was shutting down my emotional side and relating to him in a very logical, linear way."

"While covering my right eye (left brain, analytical) at work, I received a phone call requiring me to calculate hotel rates and totals for a prospective guest. Under a time pressure, I finally had to remove the patch in order to do the math involved."

"In a safe workshop environment, I patched my right eye (left brain), then did a sharing exercise with another participant. As the exercise progressed, I was more aware than usual of my emotions and need for 'personal space.' "

CLEARING BLOCKS TO VISION

This is the last exercise you will be sharing with your partner. In this one, you will be doing a visualization process to eliminate or reduce any emotional or mental blocks to seeing clearly, as well as culling any limiting beliefs or decisions that are involved. Because of the close connection between the eyes, seeing and the brain, vision may be improved by a change in perspective, making more positive decisions or resolving some old emotional issue.

Much of seeing is controlled by the autonomic nervous system, and is therefore controlled by the unconscious mind. This visualization process engages the unconscious mind, enlisting it in making changes. The process also gets the conscious mind and the unconscious mind to work together, increasing rapport between "head and heart," intellect and habit.

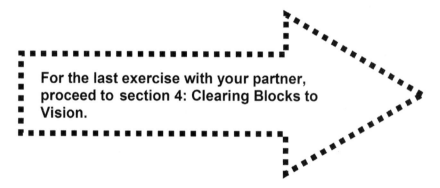

For the last exercise with your partner, proceed to section 4: Clearing Blocks to Vision.

RECHECK YOUR VISION

Now it is time to re-check your vision one last time to see if there has been an improvement. If you see an improvement, congratulations! If you see no improvement or even a slight worsening, don't be concerned. Remember the gym exercises and Pete Cisco's theory that improvement happens *after* the exertion during the recovery period.

You may be wondering whether vision can actually be improved. A list of a few groups that have training programs to improve vision from normal to beyond may provide an incentive for you to do Eye Yoga.

- Pilots for the U.S. Air Force and many commercial airlines.

- Athletic teams, like the N.Y. Yankees and the Dallas Cowboys.

- Athletes like Virginia Wade (tennis champion) and Val Skinner (golf pro).

- Connecticut State Police.

VISION IMPROVEMENT COMMENTS AND CONTROVERSIES

Not every optometrist subscribes to the idea that one can improve their eyesight with eye exercises. Considering the history of optics, that is not entirely surprising. Optics is the only field that has ever claimed to be a closed field. Opticians from the 1940s and 1950s thought there was nothing more to discover in the field of optics. Many were proud of the fact that they knew everything that could be known and theirs was the only closed science. In the field today, some of this influence may still linger in limited belief systems about what is possible. Fortunately, many in the field of optometry in our modern times have expanded both their treatments as well as their beliefs. Some offices at least contain vision therapy centers and alternative treatments, such as colored light therapy.

Originally, corrective lenses were designed to correct the eyeballs. You might be given a set of glasses to wear for several days, then a weaker set for another few, and so on until your eyes improved, and all the trainer glasses would be returned to the doctor. Now, you are sold a pair of glasses that you keep until your eyes either get better or worse, at which time you are sold a new pair. Usually, eyes continue to decline in acuity with constant use of glasses. The limiting belief is that our eyes deteriorate with age, and that it is a natural progression we can expect.

Having come this far in the book, you may have experienced an improvement in your eyesight, however great or small, whether temporary or lasting. This means that there is a connection between eye exercises and your vision. It means that you can get your brain to talk to your eyes in order to get them to see more clearly. It also means that once you understand how you are seeing, you can expand your thinking to improve your vision. You can allow yourself to expand your experience of the world in a visual, auditory or kinesthetic way, and in a right- or left-brained way, depending on which functions you may have been shutting down or have chosen to de-emphasize. By patching, you can encourage the less-engaged eye and corresponding brain functions to become stronger and participate more fully in your vision and your life.

SECTION TWO

EYE-BRAIN PHYSIOLOGY

CHAPTER 11

EYE-BRAIN DEVELOPMENT

EMBRYONIC DEVELOPMENT

As early as the first month of embryonic development, the brain has two button-shaped discs or eye buds on either side. As the fetus grows and the eye buds move around to the front of the head, they extend externally as the skull develops. *Gray's Anatomy* (Henry Gray) describes this process: "The optic nerve and the retina are developed as an outgrowth from the rudimentary brain, which extends toward the side of the head ..." (p. 1180). The optic nerve arises as a hollow outgrowth of the brain, eventually becoming solid. As the retina forms, the optic nerve fibers grow backward along the optic stalk to the brain, converting to a solid optic nerve. From this, one can see that the eyes are literally an external extension of the brain.

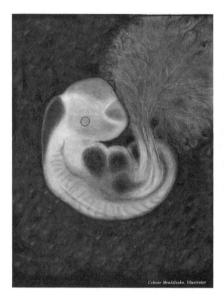
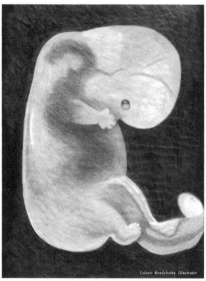

Celeste Mendelsohn, Illustrator

PHYSIOLOGY OF THE EYE

To understand your eyes, a brief review of their physiology will help give a "map" or schemata to follow. Your eyeball is filled with vitreous "jelly" and is protected by a thick sheath around it called the "sclera." In the back of the eyeball, the surface of the sclera is connected to the tough outer covering of the "optic nerve," the cable that links the eyes and the brain. At the front of the eyeball is a transparent porthole called the "cornea," through which you can see the "iris" and the pupil. The cornea has five layers and its shape is supposedly fixed. More than a window, it is a converging lens, bending light rays and focusing them to the back of the inside of the eye onto the retina. The cornea does about three-fourths of the focusing work.

The iris is made of connective tissue, muscles and pigmentation that give it color. Brown eyes have a lot of pigment whereas blue eyes have very little. The iris regulates the size of the "pupil," the hole in the center of the iris that lets in light to the retina. The iris opens and closes the pupil like the f-stop on a camera—wider in the dark and constricted in bright light. Tucked behind the iris is the "elastic lens," about the size and shape of an M&M® candy. It is responsible for about one-quarter of the focusing work. The cornea has fixed focus power, while the lens has variable focus power. The lens is held in place by ciliary muscles, which tighten or relax to change the lens shape by flattening or rounding it.

DRAWINGS OF THE EYE

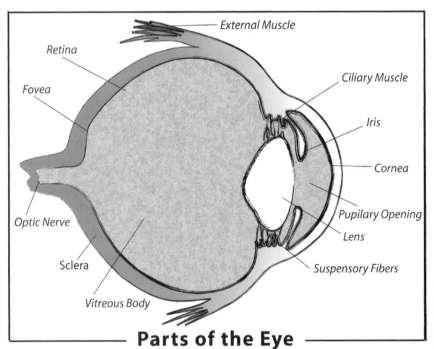

External Muscle

Retina

Fovea

Ciliary Muscle

Iris

Cornea

Optic Nerve

Pupilary Opening

Lens

Sclera

Suspensory Fibers

Vitreous Body

Mendelsohn, Illustrator

Parts of the Eye

The light-sensitive "retina" is located on the inside back of the eyeball's sclera. It is the reason for having all of the rest of the eyeball's apparatus. Not only does it register the image observed, it also breaks the image down into countless elements, such as brightness, color, position, angles and movement. It encodes them into electrical/chemical signals that are transmitted via ganglion cells to the brain through a collection of nerve fibers called the "optic nerve." According to Liberman (*Light: Medicine of the Future,* p. 20), they are sent to the brain at approximately 234 miles per hour!

The retinal discrimination falls into three categories:

- Light Discrimination – brightness discrimination, color.

- Spatial Discrimination – recognition of shape or pattern, pattern-maker, form recognition, brain fills in the missing pieces. C λ T is seen as CAT by the brain, which changes the λ to an A to make the familiar word CAT.

- Temporal Discrimination – time varying stimuli like flickering lights. The brain will not see the flickering picture in a TV, but will make it one continuous picture, for example. Recent research theorizes that the spatio-temporal discriminations cannot be separated. Movement and location in space are inextricably linked.

The light rays of the image we are seeing are imprinted on the retina upside down and reversed. The retina converts the photoelectric image into countless codings, like computer data bits, which are then sent electrically and chemically to the brain. In other words, what eventually gets to the brain is not at all the image we are seeing. The brain gets many data bits that it will then choose to ignore (delete), make into something familiar or expected (distort), or categorize and make a conclusion about (generalize). (See chapter 22 for more information on this).

- Delete: It is not important or you don't want to see it, so the brain acts as if it did not see it. The brain only pays attention to what it thinks is important. We've all had someone ask if we noticed something of which we were oblivious.

- Distort: You see a familiar face in a crowd that reminds you of someone, only to discover it is a stranger that has reminded you of your friend.

- Generalize: You make a generalization from one event. You miss several tennis balls and conclude that not only are you having a bad day, but you are a really poor tennis player.

The retina has a central point of highest sensitivity and keenest vision called the "fovea." The retina contains photosensitive brain cells called rods and cones. Each eye has 137 million photoreceptors, 130 million of which are rods and 7 million are cones. The rods see black and white, shades of gray and shading, and gross shapes; they also allow us to see in dim light and give us our "peripheral vision." They are spread out on the sides of the retina. The cones see colors, fine visual acuity needed for close work and detect small objects and details. They need plenty of light to see. They give "central vision." Most cones are packed in and close to the fovea, a tiny spot near the center of the retina where the image is focused by the lens. This means that we should clearly see the one spot we're focusing on, and everything else around it will be proportionally not as clear depending on its distance away. The less-clear peripheral vision lets us know where we are in space, providing spatial and size concepts.

The "muscles" involved in seeing are:

- The extraocular muscles that turn the eyeball.
  - Any one eye movement may involve all six muscles to some degree.
  - Their functions are complex and not isolated.

- The tiny ciliary muscles that adjust the lens.
  - They shape (round or flatten) the lens to adjust the refraction.
  - The intent is to get the image to land on the fovea.
  - How this is done and how we see is complex.
  - They are controlled by the autonomic nervous system, responsible for functions like heart rate and digestion. This means you aren't consciously aware of these non-voluntary functions (e.g., suppressing or shutting off vision in one eye). With the feedback from vision exercises, you can increase your awareness so that the brain can learn how to use these muscles and your eyes most efficiently.

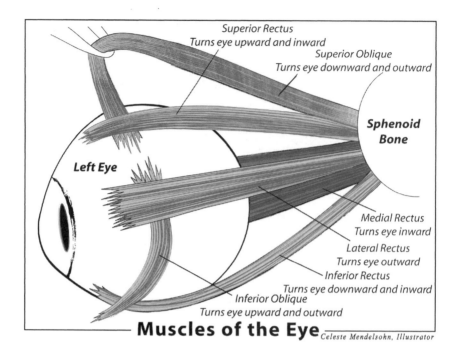

Superior Rectus
Turns eye upward and inward

Superior Oblique
Turns eye downward and outward

Sphenoid Bone

Left Eye

Medial Rectus
Turns eye inward

Lateral Rectus
Turns eye outward

Inferior Rectus
Turns eye downward and inward

Inferior Oblique
Turns eye upward and outward

Muscles of the Eye
Celeste Mendelsohn, Illustrator

There are several functions of the muscles that are important in good vision. One is to keep the eyes moving flexibly. Some sight is turned off when there is no movement. The glassy stare seen when "there's nobody home" is an indication that the person is not really seeing. The other is to keep the eye muscles relaxed and flexible. While one muscle pulls, the other lets go. Both actions are needed, so both sides of the brain need to be engaged. If one pulls all the time, you can get a turned eye. If both pull all the time, you may get farsightedness. One theory, espoused by Bates in particular, purports that if the oblique muscles wrap too tightly around the eye, it can cause nearsightedness. (This theory is not accepted by many in the field).

"Nerves that regulate eye movements work closely with the portion of the brain that governs consciousness by acting as sensory filters."

—Jacob Liberman, *Take Off Your Glasses and See*

CHAPTER 12

THE VISION PROCESS

The relationship of eye movements to thinking starts early in life. The baby begins its relationship with space at birth and learns how to use its eyes by moving toward or away from mother, food, sounds and toys. At first, the baby may use each eye separately, but soon learns to use the eyes together as it learns to creep, crawl, walk and run. If the baby learns to use both eyes together, then depth perception develops. If not, the brain may compensate and switch off the vision in one eye to avoid the confusion of seeing double.

Now let's look at what happens when we see something. Light is energy, emitted in waves or rays, usually in a straight line. Light bounces off of an image and goes to the eyes. Like taking a picture with a camera, light is needed to see. In order to provide a sharp image on the retina, in the back of the eyeball, these light rays must be bent (refracted) by the cornea and lens to focus the image onto the retina. But the eye works like a camera, again—like the image on the film negative, the image made on the retina is *upside down and reversed*! It is then up to the brain to unscramble it and make sense out of it.

When light hits the cornea, it is refracted—turned upside down and reversed. Then it comes to the lens, where the front of the lens rights it. But then the back of the lens refracts it back to upside down and reversed again. When the retina sends encoded signals to the brain, the brain somehow makes the images right-side up and un-reversed again.

Not only that, each eye is seeing the image from a slightly different perspective and place. These two images are integrated into one by the brain as well. This gives us clear central vision and depth perception!

If you hold a pencil out in front of you and then close one eye and then the other in rapid succession, alternating back and forth, you should see the pencil and the background objects appear to jump back and forth in space. This is because your eyes are several inches apart and in a spatially different place. This means each eye sees the image from a slightly different perspective.

Now here's something curious. When each eye is seeing totally different images, the brain often doesn't seem to be able to integrate the images. For example, you can hold up a barrier to your nose so each eye can only see on its side. Then show each eye a different image, maybe a green dot to one and a red dot to the other, or a red ten of hearts to one and a black ace of spades to the other. In this case, the brain will resolve the dilemma in one of several ways. It may alternate back and forth from one image to the other, from left to right eye images. Or it may suppress one image and "see" only the other. In an experiment where one eye was shown a pattern of horizontal lines and the other eye was shown a pattern of vertical lines, the brain made a mosaic patchwork of horizontal and vertical swatches. It was unable to integrate the two dissimilar images, so it created partial images of each.

Left Eye View + Right Eye View = What Both Eyes See as Fused Image

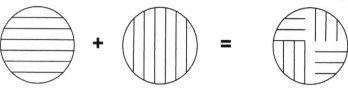

That is still not all. You may know that the left side of the brain typically controls the right side of the body and the right brain side typically controls the left side of the body. In the eyes, however, *each eye* sends half its image to the right brain and the other half to the left brain. Imagine the eyeball's vision field divided in half. You have the nasal half, nearest the nose, and the temporal half, nearest the temple. Remembering that the image on the retina is reversed, the nasal half of the eye sends its image to the temporal hemifield of the retina, and the temporal half of the eye sends its image to the nasal hemifield of the retina. Then, the nasal retina image crosses over to the opposite side of the brain, while the temporal side of the retina stays on the same side of the brain.

"This splitting and crossing reorganizes the retinal outputs so that the left hemisphere processes information from the right visual field and the right hemisphere processes information from the left visual field."

—www.cog.brown.edu/courses/cgooo1/lectures/visualpaths.html

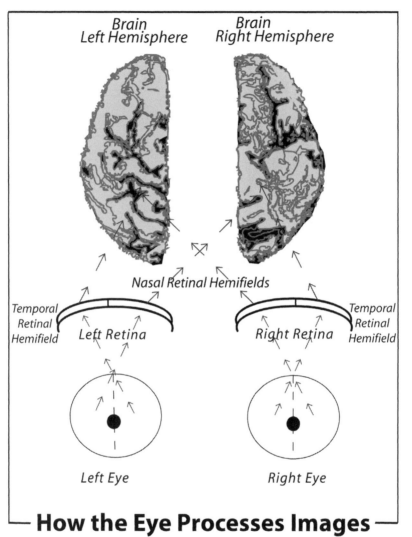

Celeste Mendelsohn, Illustrator

How the Eye Processes Images

Many vision professionals report one eye having a very different personality than the other eye, in terms of how it processes information. Our personal experiences, and those of clients and workshop participants, also bear this out. Usually, the right eye processes in a left-brain way, and the left eye processes in a right-brain way. Vision therapist, Suzan Dallé, found it to be an 80/20 split with, for example, the right eye processing 80% in a left-brain way. Readers will want to check this out for themselves.

Which eye processes emotionally? Which eye is more logical? Which eye is more right-brained? Which eye is more left-brained?

- Think of something highly emotional. First, cover your right eye, then cover your left eye as you do this. With which eye is the emotion stronger? One eye may think logically about the situation, while the emotions may be felt more strongly with the other eye.

- Most people find looking with their left eye is more emotional, and looking with their right eye is more logical.

- Continue to experiment to see which of your eyes processes mostly in a right-brain way and which processes mostly in a left-brain way.

One physiological explanation of why each eye seems to have a different personality, despite sending its information to both sides of the brain, has to do with the nose. Because the nose blocks part of the nasal side of the visual field, this would make the temporal field larger. Therefore, more of the right eye's vision is sent to the left brain, and more of the left eye's vision is sent to the right brain. Special thanks to Dr. Neal Apple, M.D., who offered this possible explanation. The truth is that we do not really know how we are able to see. We still don't totally understand the process of eye-to-brain processing that results in "vision."

Optometrist and author Roberto Kaplan delves deeper as he talks about the right and left eye personalities in his article, "Light, Lenses and The Mind – The Potent Medicine of Optometry." "Clinical experience in vision therapy reveals that each eye input carries a particular energetic charge that is needed for the development of high-level integration. I began tracking which eye the myopic patient was more prone to suppress and correlated this to the preferred eye and information gathered during the case history. From these, and other patching experiments, it appears that each eye carries its own family history and story about the survival personality." He views the integration of the inputs of the right and left eyes to be like the relationship between man and woman.

Dr. Fred Schiffer, a psychiatrist on the faculty at Harvard Medical School, has developed a non-standard technique for awakening and releasing emotional troubles or traumas. Believing that the two sides of the brain house separate and distinct personalities, he restricts vision input to only one side of the brain via special goggles (covering one side and the nasal half of the other side), to be able to talk to that side of the brain. He switches the goggles to cover the other side and to allow the two sides to dialogue with each other, with reported therapeutic successes.

When working with a client who was unable to break her addictive attraction to a partner, I had her regress to a past life with this person, where she first lost herself in giving everything to him, while he continued to treat her badly. On a whim, I asked her to imagine herself in this past life closing her left eye and viewing the situation. Imaginally using her right eye, she clearly saw that he was taking advantage of her. She could see her obsessive pattern and decided to walk away from the relationship. I then had her imagine viewing the situation with her left eye, in her mind closing her right eye. She immediately went back into the sticky, addictive emotional attachments. The point is that even when she was *imagining* closing one eye in an *imagined* past life, the right- and left-brain processing differences were clearly manifested in this client's experiences.

Let's go back into physiology to complete the vision journey, this time from the retina and optic nerve to the various parts of the brain. There is a giant "relay race" from the retina's rods and cones, to bipolar cells, to ganglion cells, down the optic nerve, consisting of about one million axons. About 80% of these axons go to a junction box in the brain, called the Lateral Geniculate Nucleus (LGN). Here each ganglion axon releases a neurotransmitter that passes its bit of visual message to another neuron that takes it on to the visual cortex in the back of the brain. The retinal neurons detect contrast changes within an image as well as edges and shadows. The LGN, deep in the center of the brain, separates retinal inputs into two streams: 1) color and fine structure, and 2) contrast and motion.

A newborn baby's visual cortex has many haphazard connections that must be pruned and reduced to improve their ability to see fine detail and recognize patterns and shapes. Gradually, the baby's visual cortex is taught to see the red of a red rose under many different gradations of illumination, teaching what red means. This is, by the way, strongly influenced by what color a person expects an object to be. In fact, almost all higher order features of vision are influenced by expectations based on past experience. We literally teach ourselves to see what we expect to see. For example, when flashed a card with a red ace of spades, a person will often report seeing a red ace of hearts or a black ace of spades. While we can be fooled, as in optical illusions or seeing what we expect to see, this gives us the ability to see and respond to the visual world very quickly!

The other 20% of the optic nerve axons get shunted directly to the more autonomic portions of the brain that control things such as pupil size—pupils close down in bright light and open up in dim light—and coordination of eye/head movements necessary to track a moving object. They also create and stitch together a series of still images called "saccades" to make a scan of a visual landscape appear smooth instead of a blur. You can actually see the eye make these tiny "saccade" jumps as a person scans a view.

Lest we get lulled into thinking that the eyes are only for eyesight, let's examine another function that the light-to-electrical impulses have. Not only are they sent to the visual cortex to construct "images" of what we see, some also travel to the *hypothalamus*, the brain's "master control." Here the light taken in from our eyes affects our body's regulatory centers, our circadian rhythms, our hormones (melatonin, for example), our endocrine and nervous systems.

Light energy is sent directly to the hypothalamus, which coordinates and regulates most of our life-sustaining functions, such as activity and sleep, growth, reproduction and emotions. The hypothalamus directs the pituitary gland secretions, which regulates the body's endocrine system and the chemical hormonal messengers being constantly secreted and readjusted. These affect such things as our thyroid, adrenals, reproductive organs, kidneys and growth of long bones, muscles and internal organs (Liberman, *Light: Medicine of the Future,* p. 22–27). According to Liberman, even the ancient Greeks believed that light to the eyes was the most accessible path to the body's internal organs. The portion of our nervous system that is responsible for balancing rest and activity is the Autonomic Nervous System, the ANS, which has two subsystems, the sympathetic (action, movement) and the parasympathetic (rebuilding, rest, rejuvenation). The ANS also receives its orders from the hypothalamus, which gets light energy from our eyes.

Technically we do not "see" with our eyes. As stated earlier, what the eyes see is not imprinted or copied exactly onto the brain. Rather, the eyes participate as an input device in the visual experience. The brain constantly categorizes stimuli, sorting experiences into probable meanings and predictabilities, paying attention to differences and to movement. Otherwise, we would be overwhelmed with too much information, like the experience of an infant as described by William James, as a "blooming, buzzing, confusion." In this way, vision is constructed in the brain with the help of the input from our eyes. When we are driving and see, for example, a "No Paking" sign, our brain will fill in the missing letter, so we "see" what we expect: "No Parking."

"Although most people are born with the potential to see, vision itself is learned. We learn to interpret the light falling on the retina. Most of this learning occurs naturally before age six."

—D. L. Cook, O.D., (*What Every Pilot Needs to Know,* p. 76)

The brain can actually alter the input from the retina. Pribram and Spinelli demonstrated in various experiments that the way stimuli (afferent inputs) are received can be changed from moment to moment by the motor output (efferent) system of the brain. The brain selects its input, which is correlated with the body's muscle movements and motor output (Ornstein, *The Psychology of Consciousness*, p. 60–61). In an experiment with kittens who were allowed a mere three hours of light a day, only the kittens who were allowed to walk around during that time developed normal vision. The passive kittens could hardly see (Ornstein, p. 62).

Caribbean natives could not see the ships of Christopher Columbus on the horizon as they approached. They had no experience, concept or belief to make what they saw believable. Their eyes literally "suppressed" the vision of the ships, until a shaman, using other senses, brought to awareness what was happening.

(Taken from the 2004 film, "What the Bleep Do We Know!?")

Other studies, particularly those by Wilder Penfield, M.D. (Wilder Penfield, p. 303), have shown that vision can be experienced by electrically stimulating various parts of the brain. Patients would have whole-cloth memories of past events, seeing them as if they were actually there when he poked a certain part of their brain. Vision can also be internally constructed by daydreaming, hypnosis and visualizations. Sometimes these seem to have a life of their own, as real as if we were actually seeing them with our eyes instead of our brain. Visions and hallucinations may also be induced by high fever, sensory deprivation, fasting and drugs.

We can conclude from these examples that vision is constructed by the brain. The point being made is that our eyes are not a stand-alone mechanical device like a camera. They are closely entwined with our brain and motor functions. The brain can neurologically block from view what you don't believe or distort what you see in order to fit what you do believe. In addition, they have direct access to the master control gland, the hypothalamus, which controls most of our bodily, health and life-sustaining functions.

"Nature gets credit which in truth should be reserved for ourselves, the rose for its scent, the nightingale for his song, and the sun for its radiance. The poets are entirely mistaken. They should address their lyrics to themselves and should turn them into odes of self congratulations on the excellence of the human mind..."

—Alfred North Whitehead

CHAPTER 13

THE IRIS AS A REFLECTION OR MAP

IRIDOLOGY—DIAGNOSTIC MEDICINE

Everything that has happened to your body is mirrored in your eyes. Eye doctors regularly examine the retina for early signs of health problems in the body like hypertension and diabetes. The sclera (white of the eye) also gives indications about the body's health. Interestingly, the connection between the eyes, the mind and the body is so close that the blood pressure in the brain can be measured through the interocular pressure! The iris gives a printout of everything that is going on in the body. In fact, there is a whole branch of diagnostic medicine called Iridology, which reads the iris, the pupil and the whites of the eyes for physiological conditions and irregularities.

Iridology was first established in the mid-nineteenth century by a Hungarian physician, Ignatz von Peczely. The story goes that he had a pet owl that had broken its leg. In looking sympathetically into the owl's eyes, he noticed a small dot on the iris just under the pupil. He never forgot that, and years later, as a physician, he noticed that every patient with a broken leg had a corresponding dot on the iris in the same place as the owl's. He eventually found relationships between the vital organs and the eyes, where changes in the organs showed in the iris. Iridology was developed in greater detail by Peter Johannes Thiel, a German scientist, and more recently by the late Dr. Bernard Jensen, D.C., N.D., from Escondido, California.

It is based on the idea that since the iris contains a myriad of nerve endings, it can be used as a barometer for body changes. The iris is sectioned into minute areas corresponding to the body's internal organs, skeleton, musculature and body functions. According to Dr. Jensen, the eyes reveal structural defects, latent toxic settlements, latent inherent weaknesses in organs, anemia, drug poisonings, chemical imbalances, and the power to get well! (Deimel, *Vision Victory Via Vital Foods, Visual Training & Vitamins*, p. 105)

INNATE PERSONALITY TRAITS REFLECTED IN THE IRIS

As early as infancy, certain personality traits can be detected in people. Certainly our upbringing and our environment help shape us enormously, yet often certain innate tendencies are clearly distinguishable early on. A child may love to be held, to be physically active, like to touch things and learn by doing (kinesthetic). Another may have an ear for music and language, love songs, rhythm and dance, and go quickly to sleep when a lullaby or story is heard (auditory). One child wants to know how things work and gravitates toward intellectual, left-brained activities. Another just wants to play ball and sports or shows a high degree of intuition, loving artistic expressions, which are more right-brained activities. Your iris contains an intricate array of configurations and markings that are a physical map of your personality.

The link between the markings and patterns in the iris and a person's innate personality and emotional traits was developed by Denny Ray Johnson, a highly intuitive and spiritual man. He says that much of a person's personality has to do with the way they process and respond to sensory information, (the senses of sight, sound, touch, feelings, etc.). He declares that the iris, a kind of "blueprint of inheritance," is the genetic representation of the DNA transmission at conception. In his book, *What the Eye Reveals*, he says that the iris reflects much more than just the personality; it reflects the person's "…life potential, revealing character strengths and aspects of the personality that are undeveloped."

Over the years, Johnson gathered these repeated themes and developed the Rayid Method. The purpose of the Rayid Method is to "balance physical, emotional and mental systems in order to become more sensitive to your true self" (Johnson, p. 7). He began teaching this method of diagnosis to various clinicians including osteopathic and medical physicians, healing practitioners, eye doctors and nurses. Roberto Kaplan, skeptical at first, has found this method to be accurate at least 80% of the time with his optometric clients.

> "Each constitutional structure is a standing wave pattern in the physical vehicle of the body, just like the pattern light makes in a droplet of vibrating water…We each have a different frequency of vibration, a different pattern…Each of us is unique."
>
> —Denny Ray Johnson, *What the Eye Reveals* (p. 6)

Johnson came up with four primary iris structures, which he related to specific personality profiles. They are: Jewel for visual and thoughts, Flower for auditory and emotions, Stream for kinesthetic and feelings, and Shaker for the moving power of awakening and change. By looking at the fibers and forms of the iris, one can predict certain tendencies with which a person was born. In other words, we can all develop skills in using our five senses through practice and experience. The idea that we are born with certain innate tendencies that are reflected in the formations of the irises in the eyes gives pause for reflection. If this is accurate, it would mean one more link between the eyes, the brain and the person's unique traits.

John Meluso, in his book, *eyeTALK*™, builds on Johnson's work, calling the four eye patterns: Visual, Auditory, Kinesthetic, and Haptic, corresponding to the different learning and communication styles of Neuro-Linguistic Programming. NLP has the predominant learning and processing styles of visual, auditory, kinesthetic, and a fourth category, auditory-digital (an analytical, evaluative style). Meluso, like Johnson, adds a fourth category to the iris patterns called Haptic, similar to Johnson's Shaker. (It is unclear whether Haptic is in any way similar to NLP's digital type). Each of these patterns indicates some common personality behaviors, for which the eyes are a visual aid. They indicate the person's "native language," from which they can branch out and learn other languages (skills).

Becoming aware of your own innate characteristics, as well as those of people with whom you communicate, can be a delightful and illuminating skill. You can understand why one person may stand very close to others when speaking or listening, while another keeps backing up from such close proximity. You can predict who will respond to touch, who needs to know all about your background before warming up to you, who feels the "vibes" of a room instantly and who responds to the tone of voice more than the words spoken. Following is a brief description of each type for you to experiment with.

1. Visual

The iris of the visual has straight fibers dotted with gold or brown pigment flecks. Below is a planar depiction of what one would see in the fibers or lines in the wheel of the iris.

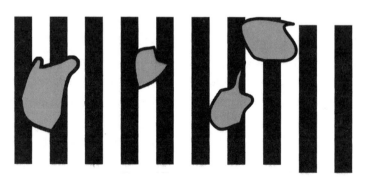

The characteristics of a Visual person are:

Analytical

Thinking

Visual

Initially reserved upon meeting someone new

Interested in a person's qualifications, background, family and data

Stands symmetrically with weight equally distributed, often with arms folded

Doesn't like a lot of touch, especially initially

Will stand at a slightly farther distance from someone than other types

2. Auditory

The iris of the Auditory person has curved or rounded openings in the fibers, like petals or curtains being parted.

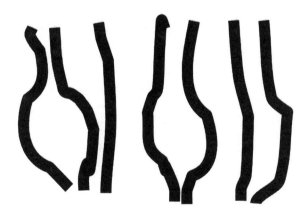

The characteristics of an Auditory person are:

Emotional, feeling

Auditory

Likes sequence

Rhythmic, whether in daily routines or musically

Easily senses feelings, yet doesn't hold onto them as long as a kinesthetic person; able to let them go more easily

Usually flexible, spontaneous

Sociability and rapport skills

Responds to tone of voice more than the words spoken

3. Kinesthetic

The iris of the Kinesthetic person has straight fibers, similar to those of a Visual person's but without the dots.

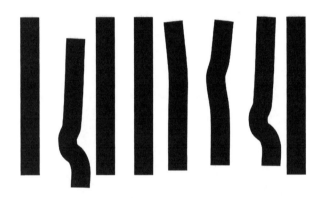

The characteristics of a Kinesthetic person are:

Intuitiveness

Sensitive—can immediately sense the "energy" in a room

Has a hard time letting go of emotions and feelings picked up

Grounded, calm

Tends to stand closer to a person with whom they are talking

Usually likes touch, unless they don't like the energy of a person

Feels comfortable in conversation when you touch their arm or shoulder

Tends to be a slower-paced thinker and speaker

A high, fast voice communication tends to be harder for them to listen to

Often is quite physical, both in learning style and communication

4. Haptic

The iris of a Haptic person may have the fibers of a Visual, Auditory or Kinesthetic person, with some rounded openings. There is always at least one dot-like pigment and usually up to three, whether in one or both eyes.

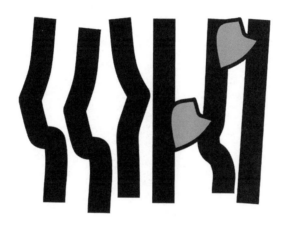

The characteristics of a Haptic person are:

Highly motivated, in motion

Good starter of projects and ideas, not necessarily a good completer

May appear almost driven, with high energy

Processes visual, auditory and kinesthetic all at the same time, which makes them seem a bit frenetic or overwhelmed at times, similar to ADD (Attention Deficit Disorder) children. Other times, they have learned to be calm on the outside, and have learned to handle that sense of having everything come into them all at once.

Originality, vitality, zeal, sometimes unpredictable

Achievement-oriented

If you are now ready to try your hand at identifying which type a person is by examining their irises, a magnifying glass with a light is a great help. If not available, use good light or a flashlight to see the iris fibers. Here are an artist's renditions of the four different types:

VISUAL:

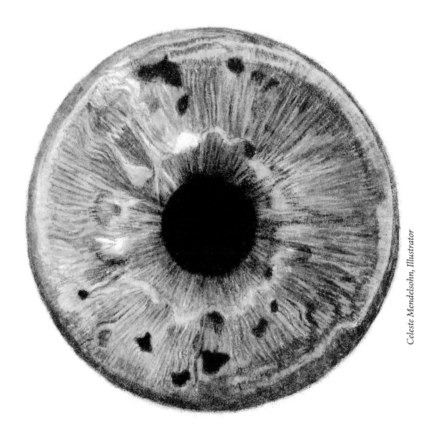

Celeste Mendelsohn, Illustrator

AUDITORY:

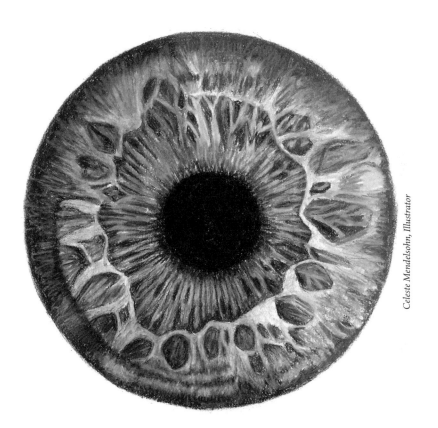

Celeste Mendelsohn, Illustrator

KINESTHETIC:

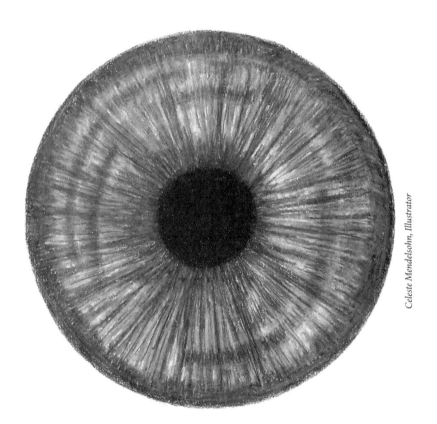

Celeste Mendelsohn, Illustrator

HAPTIC:

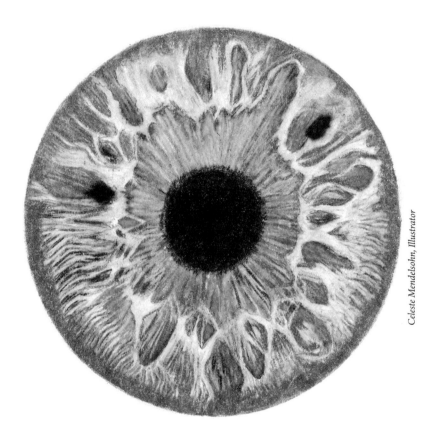

Celeste Mendelsohn, Illustrator

There are more characteristics that can be "read" in the irises, such as right- and left-brained dominance, emotional predispositions, qualities of wanting to please people, determination and rigidity. Roberto Kaplan uses iris analysis to give insight into his patients and their sight limitations. We have given a very superficial summary of the four personality types here. For those who are interested, more information can be found in the following references:

eyeTalk™: Beyond Communication to Connection by John Meluso, Jr.

What the Eye Reveals by Denny Ray Johnson and J. Erik Ness

Conscious Seeing by Robert Michael Kaplan

CHAPTER 14

SEEING EYE TO EYE

Since section 2 contains quite an eclectic array of topics, let's look at the main points made, their relationship to each other, and some possible meanings. First, in chapter 11, we see that the eyes and the brain are one "organ." The brain extends itself externally by way of the eyes and their tethers, the optic nerves. We begin to see that vision is not a stand-alone process, but is integrally related to our motor skills, such as balance, eye-hand-body coordination and "where we are" in relationship to the world. Spatially, we see our position relative to everything else. We use peripheral vision for balance and movement, and we use central or foveal vision to see details.

In chapter 12, we begin to follow the three-step process of making sight into meaning or understanding. The visual image, made up of light rays, is first deposited on the retinal photosensitive cells. The retinal image, reversed and inverted, is translated into myriad different electro-chemical codes that are sent to the back of the brain by way of the optic nerve. Each eye sends half its image to one side of the brain and the other half to the other side. In addition, each eye seems to have its own personality, corresponding to the right or left side of the brain. Once the retinal image is translated into many coded signals, these signals ricochet around the brain, back and forth like bullets in a steel box. Despite scientists' best efforts to break this down, no one really understands exactly how we are able to see.

Some codes go directly to the autonomic parts of the brain, which automatically react to light and movement, adjusting our reactive responses, our neurotransmitters, hormones and peptides. For example, feedback is sent to the pupils to dilate or constrict them and eye/head movements associated with visually tracking moving objects are coordinated. You automatically run away from a lion that has jumped out at you, without having to think, "Oh, a lion. I might be in danger. I better run." That would be much too late! Some codes are sent directly to the master controlling hypothalamus and other hormone-regulating parts.

We still have not interpreted or understood what we are seeing. Most of the information is sent to the visual cortex and then forwarded to the cerebral cortex. The right brain interprets the information spatio-contextually, while the left brain looks for specifics. The brain deletes, distorts and generalizes the information in order to make sense of it.

We don't pay attention to what doesn't seem important or interesting. We also fill in information in order to quickly grasp the whole. As an example, good readers do not read every word, yet they grasp the whole meaning.

What we interpret from this is filtered by our previous experiences, memories, beliefs, language, personality traits and many other factors. These filters determine what we pay attention to. Out of this, we fabricate a personal vision of what we think is reality. Seeing is really a complex and subjective process!

In chapter 13, we find that the eyes are a micro-reflection of our whole person. The body's physical and emotional conditions, along with changes it goes through, can be "read" in the iris. This includes the person's power to get well! In addition, many innate personality traits and preclusions toward certain emotions can be detected in the iris. The iris is a map of our personality traits we were born with, our predilection toward certain behaviors and emotions.

Because the eyes are hardwired into the brain and are literally an extension of the brain, it would be a mistake to treat them as mechanical sight-producers. They are organs for creating our internal reality. They are filters for information and maps of our body health and personality. Our eyes have 70% of the body's sense receptors and are the entry point for 90% of all information we learn in our life (Liberman, *Take Off Your Glasses and See,* p. 17). They are the avenue for bringing light energy to our master control gland, the hypothalamus, which regulates a multitude of life-sustaining functions. They even give off energy at times, as windows to our soul. The eyes become the projected image of the consciousness of the personality behind them.

SEEING AND THINKING

CHAPTER 15

SIGHT AND BRAIN CONNECTION

"You can't see differently until you think differently."

—Suzan Dallé

Our eyes, hardwired into our brain, reflect how we are thinking. Even our language expresses this connection. When we feel angry, we "see red." When we are fearful, we get "tunnel vision." We can be "happy in wide-eyed wonder" or "see the world through rose-colored glasses." We can be "blind with rage," have "green-eyed jealousy," or "lose sight of an objective." We can be "blind-sided" by something or even "lose sight of objectivity" as a result of strong emotions.

El Greco supposedly had astigmatism. When the elongated figures in his paintings are viewed through glasses that correct for a certain degree of astigmatism, they appear normal instead of elongated. The poet, John Keats, who wrote "Ode on a Grecian Urn," was supposedly nearsighted, which fits with his focus on the details of the urn. On the other hand, the poet Shelley, thought to be farsighted, dealt with far visions in his works. Lord Byron was probably also farsighted because he prolifically wrote of ideas, aspirations, memories, man and nature, the past and future, the hopes of nations, and the dignity of manhood.

Dr. Jacob Liberman, in his book, *Take Off Your Glasses and See* (p. 116), reports 96% of hard-core juvenile offenders had significant vision problems. After vision therapy, their re-arrest rate dropped from 50% to 10%, and their reading skills elevated by four grade levels. There was also an increase in their self-esteem, IQ and other positive values.

Our outward behavior, our personality traits and attitudes, mirror our inward thoughts and feelings, and our inward processing affects how we see the world, both literally and figuratively. In that way, a person's eyesight limitation is one part of their psychological and behavioral profile.

Vision fitness involves much more than sight. It involves the balancing of sight and brain through your eyes, according to Kaplan, optometrist and vision education specialist. His goal is "to clear the mind's eye by shifting a person's fundamental perspective on life from a fragmentary and mechanistic one to a more holistic view" (*East West Magazine*, p. 40). Vision is more than a mechanical function to be fixed with measures such as corrective lenses or surgeries. It is an interactive result of environmental, biological and genetic conditions. It literally tells how we perceive our world. It is a window into our inner vision. Kaplan says if we balance our inner perceptions first, through personal awareness and mind-body dynamics, our life becomes more harmonious.

Remembering that the eyes are an extension of the brain, it may not then be surprising to find that there is evidence to show that the way in which we see is reflected in some of our personality traits. For example, a nearsighted person (one who sees well up close) might want more detail, may like to understand things close to them or may be fearful of the future. A farsighted person (one who has difficulty seeing up close) may get frustrated with too much detail or not want to get too involved emotionally. A presbyopic person (with age has increasing difficulty seeing up close) may be avoiding unresolved anger and want to keep emotional entanglements at bay, while seeking the big picture or "What's it all about, Alfie?" They also may not need a lot of details and facts. A person with astigmatism (uneven cornea/lens) can see many points of view, but may have a hard time making up their mind. Possibly one part of their life is incongruent with the rest of their personality or values.

Dr. Jacob Liberman, a master of one-line quotes, says:

"If the world outside is unclear, it may simply be a signal that something inside is unclear."

"Since the mind and vision are inseparable, fix vision by looking into the mind."

A client in her fifties found her near sight deteriorating (presbyopia). She described her life as becoming quite uncomfortable. She had gone through a difficult divorce and she felt the pangs of "empty nest" as her children left home. At some point she made a connection between having to hold reading material at arm's length and holding people at arm's length. She was pushing away any potential intimacy or emotional involvement. With this awareness, she was able to distinguish between the physical way she was using her eyes and her emotional need for safety. As a result, she was able to reclaim her near vision through eye exercises.

A couple came in for vision counseling. He was farsighted and she was nearsighted. From their interactions it was plain that, as much as they loved each other, there was some friction, as if they weren't speaking each other's language. I asked him if he was frustrated by her overwhelming need for information and detail. With a sigh of great relief, he emphatically agreed. He said that even when he understood the idea, she insisted on going over and over it down to the gnat's eyebrows. He had learned to tune her out in self-defense. I asked her if she felt he was emotionally unavailable and a little distant. She also emphatically agreed. She thought he never listened to her and wasn't interested in what she had to say. The more he did this, the more she tried to engage him, which seemed to make it worse. The more she went over it in detail, the more he tuned her out, because he had already gotten her point. He had little tolerance for such detail, while she felt a big-picture overview wasn't at all fulfilling.

There are advantages to being aware of the correlation between the different vision limitations and their associated traits. This information can be useful not only to you and your personal growth, but also in social and business settings, as well as with family and friends. Kaplan, in his fascinating book, *The Power Behind Your Eyes*, explores this in greater depth.

Rapport: You can use this information to create better rapport with others. It gives insight into certain personality traits of other people. Knowing how they see, you can match your communication style with their preferences, making your interchanges go more smoothly. If you know the person is farsighted, you may want to give them more global, big-picture overviews rather than bore in with too much detail. They may also prefer a little emotional distance.

Conversely, if the individual with whom you are dealing is nearsighted, they may desire quite a bit of detail before they can deal with the bigger picture. They may delight in and need close, emotional bonding. Knowing what makes another person comfortable can be particularly useful when dealing with your partner, your boss or a client. It can be applied to a variety of situations, such as sales, business, education and communication with family and friends.

"One of my sons is very, very nearsighted. Without lenses, he needs to hold things inches away from his face. I remember when he was five years old, he made a beautifully-proportioned clay elephant. While it was only 2 inches big, it had intricate detail. My other son is farsighted. As a child he was not detail-oriented. When I'd try to explain the details of something to him, once he understood the concept enough to his satisfaction, he'd reject more information, even if it meant walking away. I could have used this information in raising those boys!"

—K. J. S., Flemington, New Jersey

Alleviating the Underlying Causes to Improve Eyesight: Once you become aware of the connection between vision and emotional conditions, you can take steps to alleviate the underlying causes. If you understand the stresses, emotional dynamics and environmental situations that cause the vision limitations, you can work to eliminate or reduce them. This may involve resolving old issues and emotions, easing stresses, gaining more choices in an area, self-acceptance or forgiveness. This may apply not only to yourself, but also in raising your children and in dealing with aging parents. It also has implications for education and therapy.

Vision Flexibility: Vision is a very flexible process. Antonia Orfield (p. 130) reported many cases of Multiple Personality Disorder (MPD) where different personalities have different vision prescriptions due to the different life experiences of each personality. The implications of this suggest that vision could be context-dependent. You might be able to see clearly when needed, such as while reading a menu or driving, and return the vision to a more comfortable, fuzzy look when clarity is not needed. Being in rapport with one's unconscious mind and directing the brain to see well could allow such visual flexibility. The 2000 Nobel Prize winner in Medicine, neuroscientist Eric Kandel, explains that the structure of our brains and the degree of sensitivity in the fine connections between our nerves aren't fixed, but can be *changed by learning*, opening the possibility of recalibrating our sight. Vision flexibility could increase one's alternatives to having an overdependence on the 20/20 focus.

New Sight: Understanding the eye-mind connection has even deeper implications than understanding psychological tendencies and improving eyesight. By understanding the deeper meaning of vision, one can use the metaphor of sight to apply to a more global vision, gaining insights, seeing new possibilities and deepening spirituality. The idea would be to use our *eyesight* as a metaphor for our vision *insight* to *envision* new possibilities and create new realities.

The next chapter deals with the psychology of vision—the personality traits and emotions associated with each condition. In addition to the psychology, there are other factors that affect vision. In chapter 17, factors such as the strength of your lens prescription, nutrition, exercise, posture, hereditary factors and stress are explored. Some corollary suggestions are made for vision improvement. Chapter 18 explores the effects of light on various physical, mental and emotional functions. In chapter 19, Vision as a Metaphor, the collective power of visionary ideas and the transcendent aspects of vision are touched upon. And finally, in chapter 20, the interrelatedness of form (physical eyes) and function (vision) is looked at. Does the way you see structure your thinking or does the way you think mold and influence your eyesight?

CHAPTER 16

PERSONALITY TRAITS AND THE EMOTIONAL NATURE OF VISION

OVERVIEW

Each vision type has its own particular psychological constellation of emotions, patterns and causes. However, underlying each of these vision types is the desire, at some core psychological level, not to see. Before going into detail on some of the vision conditions, an overview is given to summarize the possible psychological characteristics of each.

Myopia/Nearsightedness

Fear-based, or trying hard not to show or admit to fears

Pulling the world in and making it smaller

Lost in thoughts and daydreams

Introversion, contraction

Analytical

Detail-oriented

Critical, judgmental

Lack of security

Trying too hard

Over-focused, tunnel vision

Straining in some way

Withdrawal from cognitive lifestyle

Need to please others

Shy, introspective

Inflexible, stubborn

Avoids confrontations with others

High stress tolerance

Farsightedness

Resentment, anger, rage

Need to be larger than self

Unresolved anger, especially from suppressed past events

Family atmosphere of high emotion

Need to distance from emotional trauma or issues

Desire to see future with clarity

Global fear or anxiety about the future

Extrovert, tending toward aggressiveness

Sometimes exhibiting behavior problems at home and school

More aware of the environment than lost in thought

Active, overactive

Presbyopia/Difficulty Seeing Up Close

Loss of flexibility

Fear of closeness, emotional pain and intimacy

Feeling a need to distance emotionally

Keeping others at arm's length

Avoiding intimacy or entanglements

State of mind—getting old

Health, activity levels deteriorating

Astigmatism

Being out of balance

Conflicting behaviors and messages

Competing emotions

Emotional chaos

Uncertainty

Tension, rigidity or twisting

Rigid, contradictory or out of balance in one area of life

Twisted spine, neck or pelvis

Tight or restricted posture

Children who changed schools often

Experiences of many family upheavals

Confusion and disorientation experienced at some time

Immigrants from very different cultures

Cataracts

Uncertainty

Inability to clarify inner thoughts

Inability to let go of "stuff"

NEARSIGHTEDNESS (MYOPIA)

This condition is where vision is clear up close, but gets blurry or unclear farther away. Physically, nearsighted people tend to lean forward as if to see things better. It is often accompanied by obvious muscle tension in their jaw, neck, shoulders, lower back and calves. Relaxing these areas helps treat the overall condition holistically.

What may be going on emotionally is a related area to consider. When the world is confusing and there is just too much going on, it is easier to pull in and deal with what can be managed. It's hard to sort through the overload and make sense of it all. So those with this condition need to limit the scope of their world, to make it more manageable. Rather than look at the whole picture, they prefer to deal with what's immediately before them in order to cope. Feeling pressured by everything, they fight off the feeling of being overwhelmed by constricting their scope. They want lots of detail about the limited scope they can handle, and strive to do that perfectly well.

By the age of five, most children have normal to slightly farsighted vision (Eulenberg, p. 1). Most nearsightedness comes on during childhood and adolescence. Sometimes nearsightedness is brought on by changing schools. In such a case, the child loses all their old friends and has to make new ones. They may have been popular before but now find different social rules. They don't know who's who and are no longer in a secure social position. That can be scary, so they just pull in their focus to what they can deal with.

Frequently nearsightedness begins around puberty. Teens don't understand the changes taking place in their bodies. They may experience intense, swinging emotions and embarrassments. People treat them differently. They may feel that they are in this nowhere-land between adulthood and childhood, where they are sometimes treated one way and sometimes expected to behave in another. Intense emotions barge in and take over. A way to deal with *all* of the changes is to pull in their world and handle that which is closer and more immediate.

Looking at the gradual progression of myopia in grade school children, the message is that seeing at a distance isn't as important as seeing up close (reading, blackboard, etc.). With so much emphasis on academic performance, the unconscious is encouraged to tune eyesight into smaller distances. A big problem with this is the emphasis on two dimensions to the sacrifice of motor involvement and spatial awareness.

When our family went on an African safari, our guide, raised to be able to see game at great distances, would point to black dots on a far hill. "See that herd of 300 eland and 200 zebra?" We could hardly see the specks much less identify the animals. So we asked him how he knew there were 300 eland. He replied, "It's simple; I count the legs and divide by four!"

There is a correlation between the academic emphasis in a society and the increase in nearsightedness (Gallop, p. 116). In the U.S., 15–25% of adults are myopic, most of whom had normal sight before age seven. However, among military academies and academic groups worldwide, myopia exceeds 50% (Eulenberg, p. 1)!

We are also encouraged to look directly at something to the exclusion of peripheral vision. Even with lenses, we must look through the optical centers to get the best optics and the least distortion. In higher prescriptions, the prismatic and spatial distortions are greater, encouraging one to move the head and neck rather than using eye movements only. This is a regression from visual development where we learn to move the eyes independently from the rest of the body! Also, in our normal environment, there is little opportunity to "stretch" our eyes by looking off into the distance, either due to time pressures and constraints or lack of visual space. This causes the eyes to be restricted to focusing close up for long periods of time, encouraging myopia.

Steve Gallop, O.D., shares his personal experience of overcoming the prevailing ideas about eyesight limiting one's ability to do other things. Being strongly nearsighted with astigmatism, he decided one day to risk riding his bicycle without any lens corrections. He rode through rush hour traffic in Philadelphia, shocked to find he did quite well, harming neither himself nor others. His helpless dependence on glasses dissolved into feeling more ability and power to control his own destiny, profoundly changing his attitude (p. 115, 117).

According to Gallop (p. 117), myopia is more than the inability to produce clear retinal images from faraway objects. He links it to a person's ability to clearly see within. Those with myopic vision frequently tend to be withdrawn and introverted. Yet their tendency to internalize their feelings may be just as distorted as their eyesight. They may tend to look to external cues as a basis for decision-making rather than trusting their inner voice, which ultimately may erode their self-esteem and widen the gap between their internal and external perceptions. If, as a nearsighted person, you use your glasses only occasionally to increase acuity for certain activities such as driving, your identity will not be affected as much as if you need to put your glasses on as soon as you get up and keep them on to function throughout the day. Even if you see the world as blurry, you need time to interact with this blurriness to understand how things are for you before accepting external correction or judgment on how things should be. You need to get to know your own "true nature" rather than simply unquestioningly accept the authority and opinions of others.

Gallop says some myopia may not be strictly optometric (p. 118). There is usually some amount of fear that accompanies it, such as fear of the unknown, fear of not being able to see clearly or fear of not being in control. Gallop overcame some of his fear by riding his bicycle without glasses. As a culture we tend to shut out our awareness of the whole in favor of honing in on the minute details. It is as if we view life through the eyepiece of a microscope rather than a wide lens.

In Kaplan's book, *Conscious Seeing*, he proposes that each eye condition gives a metaphor for a person's personality, both for their behavior and for their inner way of thinking. He came to this conclusion after interviewing tens of thousands of nearsighted patients. He encourages people to explore their present way of seeing in order to give clues to a deeper self-understanding. Genetic influences, life experiences and wearing strong prescription lenses all help to mold one's personality and behavior. In our modern world, rational thinking is encouraged. Being logical allows an individual to focus on "getting the job done" while minimizing feelings. This leads to external rewards like financial success and promotions. But by taking the time for a deeper exploration of your feelings and emotions, you can dissolve residual fears in order to develop conscious seeing. This mitigates the unbalancing effects of over-rational thinking.

Kaplan has looked at the alarming increase in nearsightedness in countries where education is emphasized. The obvious treatment of nearsightedness with prescription lenses is not reducing the prevalence of nearsightedness. His not-so-obvious approach of integrated vision therapy compares the input and output system of vision as a computer, scanner, fax and software to the interrelationship between the eye, the brain and the mind. It is his hope that combining the obvious (lenses) with the not-so-obvious (integrated vision therapy) will alleviate the nearsightedness epidemic. "It is possible that to look and see in a broader and more integrated way will help in creating a peaceful way of seeing more deeply the challenges of the world. Can this depth of perceiving into self and others lead to less need for terrorism and war?" he wonders.

ADDITIONAL FACTORS

Some contributions to myopia are extended periods of near work, habitual muscular tension and mental strain when looking at far objects.

Excessive Close Work

Myopia can also be brought on by frequent, excessive use of eyes for close-up work. After awhile, the close-work stimulus is so constant that the eyes can't relax from their contracted state. At first, people find they take longer to focus at a distance. This refocusing takes longer and longer until at some point they can no longer see far away. The tension of near work can also cut off blood supply and oxygen needed for good vision.

Mental Strain

When we focus and concentrate, we tense up. Our visual field collapses and vision contracts. This restricts absorption of new information, in a sense limiting our intelligence. Those who stutter find that it disappears when they are moving and breathing freely, as when they are singing. William Bates had a slightly different take on the cause of functional myopia. He believed that it was caused by mental strain—the (largely unconscious) effort to see the details of unfamiliar objects at a distance, objects like a blackboard or an eye chart, for example. He said that not just strain of the eye muscles, but *any* muscular activity, such as squinting, hunching the shoulders or tensing the neck, contributes to myopia. Other studies have supported him in showing that high levels of cognitive demands, e.g., solving math problems, will cause the eyes to move toward nearsightedness (Eulenberg, p. 3).

Strong Prescriptions

Most prescriptions tend to be overly strong in order to give 20/20 distance acuity. The trade-offs are fatigue and muscular tension, reduction in vision flexibility and spatial distortion. (See chapter 17).

Eyesight in Relation to Spatial Orientation

Myopia isn't just an elongation of the eyeball or a spasm. It is a reflection of the shrinking of the brain's spatial world by shrinking the peripheral vision due to stress and then by misjudgments caused by distortions from lenses (Orfield, p. 123). It can be seen in children who get progressively more nearsighted. Their spatial world shrinks to mostly central vision so they can't judge distances. The lenses warp their peripheral vision so much that their brains have to shut it out. Their eyesight continues to decline as a result of seeing clear images centrally and blurred images peripherally. They tend to shrink inward, avoiding athletic sports, bike riding and group interactions. Being poor at games and maybe being teased about their "four eyes," they spend more and more time indoors with their "noses in books." Their self-esteem and social ease begin to melt.

One of the ways to improve nearsightedness is to reprogram the brain to "see space."

"...it was a vast, mysterious and beautiful place with tunnels of deep space under the overarching trees. The light was different —more mellow—and objects were rounder and fuller. Things seemed more real...thrilling [experiences] that released a great deal of energy that had evidently been locked up in maintaining my old virtual world."

—Antonia Orfield, M.A., O.D. (p. 127)

"I remember the first day I began to see space between things. It was so beautiful! I was mesmerized by how the world looked..."

—Jane Battenberg

Many people report space being very different when they first get glasses. They aren't sure where things are any more. Sometimes the ground seems to dip away as if you are going to step into a depression. Knowing where one is in space is a mental perception of how far is far, how deep is deep and how wide is wide. Lenses are "brain-changing, brain-programming devices because they shape and control the light patterns hitting the retina and therefore the signals from the light coursing through the entire brain and influencing the entire body. They can make our vision worse or...train us to... see space differently" (Orfield, p. 125). Some optometrists help patients improve their eyesight by gradually reducing the strength of their lens prescriptions. Patients report that it seems like pushing space out with their eyes. Space expands side to side, up and down, and out to the horizon. In addition, color sensitivity increases.

It is likely that vision is really about context, balance, movement, relationship, interaction and awareness. These are usually "on automatic," controlled by the unconscious mind, yet deeply-rooted, emotionally-charged, and sensitive to change. Given this, people with myopia may experience psychological and social difficulties as well as difficulties with physical activities and sports. In dealing with the onset of blurriness, it would also be important to address the related issues of fear and control (Gallop, p. 118). Nearsighted people would do well to trust themselves and their own perceptions, relying on their internal information instead of external pressures in their decision-making. As they do the vision exercises, nearsighted people should note any emotions that may crop up. Section Four, chapter 21 gives a process to aid in dealing with emotional issues. It is also a good practice to allow a little blur in the vision. For example, I like my world a little fuzzy, and tend to see that way unless I need to sharpen my sight.

Peripheral Vision

When our sight develops, our peripheral vision develops before our central vision. When we stare directly at the detail of something, the incoming sight goes directly to the tiny fovea in the center of the retina and to the higher visual centers. The rest of the retinal fibers, comprising about 20% and covering about 80% of the retinal area, go to other areas, such as the superior colliculus, where they transmit balance, orientation, and spatial information. This is how we relate to our physical world visually. Together this means that vision is mainly a wide-angle, contextual, peripheral process with central focus added in for extra detail (Gallop, p. 119). Peripheral awareness is the first thing that is sacrificed by those with myopia when stress depletes their energy and near sight becomes all-consuming (as is the case with studying, computer work, etc.). When people are under stress, they focus their attention on what is near, stop looking at the bigger picture and stop processing peripherally.

Improving peripheral vision is very important to improving eyesight. It creates a strong basis on which to build all other areas of visual function and information processing (Gallop, p. 119). Peripheral vision gives context—the person in relationship to everything around them. As the whole becomes better understood and more usable, the parts become more meaningful and more easily grasped. Stronger lenses take away the context of the whole as the person becomes more attached to details (and to their lenses!). The idea is to get better acuity with less compensation.

Nearsightedness constricts awareness and perception, gives inefficient information for processing and problem-solving and distorts the relationship between self and environment. It can be corrected by understanding sight in relationship to the brain and to what is going on with the person. According to neuroscientist Eric Kandel, we can actually change our brain and nerve responses by learning. Meaning can actually modify the structure of the human brain. This may be employed when we tell our eyes to "sharpen up and see," telling our brains to make that blurry image clear.

Nutrition

Good nutrition is important to vision. Sugar, simple carbohydrates, not enough protein and heavily fried and refined foods can increase nearsightedness.

To change a person's nearsightedness, one has to intervene at the level of the brain program. Lenses by themselves do not do this. Learning to see space again, peripheral-awareness training, simultaneous-movement training of eyes and body, stress management and changes in mental processing all help to reprogram the brain to see.

FARSIGHTEDNESS

The farsighted person can see things at a distance clearly, but the closer the image, the less clear it is. Physically this person tends to lean back or to move things farther away from them. Looking at farsightedness as more than a physical condition, it can be seen as a communication from the brain, as if it were trying to get your attention. While nearsightedness can be an overreaction to thinking, farsightedness can be a reaction to emotions that have become too painful, as if the eyes want to keep them at arm's length. So the eyes push the vision outward into far-off space, both away from intimacy and to see into the future for clarity. Being farsighted allows a person time to prepare a response before the emotion gets closer. It gives reaction time. If a person feels like, "It's me against the world, and I need a buffer," they will either shrink their visual field (nearsighted) or push it out (farsighted). A farsighted person may also have an urge to reach outside the self, to push beyond the self to something larger, as the description of Lord Byron at the beginning of this chapter suggests. It might even be an attempt to find answers in the cosmic consciousness.

Farsightedness often accompanies a family history of strong emotions, according to Kaplan. It can be a tip-off to look within the self for old emotional wounds that need healing. Kaplan feels that the most common emotion is anger, and Gottlieb relates it to blocked rage. Kaplan recommends practicing focusing deeply on self to build an energetically strong relationship with emotions. Look inward for unresolved emotions and immature emotional patterns. Even as a farsighted person practices pulling their eyes together to see near, this may create intense feelings. Kaplan encourages his patients to focus the eyes inward, as if "crossing their eyes," for five seconds at a time. He assures that "…just for the record, your eyes cannot get stuck by crossing them inward! This is an old wives' tale." (*Conscious Seeing*, p. 196).

Doing exercises may, indeed, bring up emotions, such as anger or resentment. Rather than avoid the emotions or blame them on someone or something else, one can recognize that the emotions are there. Acknowledging the relationship between the emotions and the farsightedness also helps. The flip side of anger is passion, so anything that one can turn to with passion instead of holding in or avoiding, is a step in the right direction toward better sight.

Farsightedness is frequently accompanied by suppression, where the brain shuts off vision in one eye. Kaplan recommends practicing seeing both sides of your nose for farsighted people. If you can see both sides, then both eyes are turned on and seeing. Once the vision in both eyes has been turned on and they begin to see with depth perception, his patients describe the excitement and aliveness of seeing multidimensionally and different distances at the same time.

PRESBYOPIA OR SHORT-ARM SYNDROME

Around age forty, many people find their near sight begins to deteriorate. They find that they need to hold things farther and farther away to see the details, like trying to read a menu in a dimly-lit restaurant or a number in the phone book. While mostly affecting near vision, it can also affect distance vision. The physiological cause of presbyopia is not well-understood; it is usually thought to be the result of changes in the lens or less commonly the strength of the ciliary muscles.

This condition could relate to a build-up of unresolved emotions. This may happen during a time in their lives when elderly parents need care or pass away, children leave home, or sometimes there is a divorce. These occurrences may bring up emotions that hurt too much to deal with—emotions they'd rather push away. They don't want hurtful things to be so emotionally close. Becoming presbyopic and losing the ability to see things up close is a way of keeping an arm's distance away from pain to protect oneself from more uncomfortable experiences. In other words, their sight limitation up close reflects their need for emotional boundaries and distancing. Proximity to others may not feel particularly safe emotionally.

Presbyopia could also be attributed to reduced muscle flexibility and reduced ability to focus as well as being a result of a build-up of the repetitive demand on the eyes for near-focus activities, such as computer work, reading, writing, digital photo work, and the like. It could, however, occur at a point in life when there is no longer the need to focus on career, income, a home, children and all the demands of life that required such concentration and focus earlier. Along comes the midlife crisis, a time not so much for learning as for a more spiritual quest for life's deeper meaning, which involves far seeing. The eyes begin to reflect the inner yearnings to see the big picture, the deeper meaning, an evolution toward the spiritual.

A couple of tips to help people with presbyopia read close up without glasses may be of use. As most have already figured out, reading is easier outside on a bright day or with a bright light on the material. We find it helpful when you want to see clearly up close, without squinting or strain, to increase your peripheral vision awareness at the same time, which relaxes and clears the vision. It is a bit odd at first to be focusing on the words of a page while simultaneously being aware of the room and your surroundings, yet it seems to work well. Some notice an increased relaxation in their face, while others feel it in their eyes.

It is an accepted myth, promoted by many eye doctors, that we can expect our eyes to deteriorate as we grow older due to gradual hardening of the eye's lens. Often we accept the state of mind of "getting old." Not everyone accepts this state of mind, and there are psychological ways of changing it by remaining flexible, emotionally expressive and open to one's environment.

"At sixty five, I still don't use any lens correction or eye surgery to see up close. When I need to see better, I do a few eye yoga exercises, relax, and my eyes respond!"

—Jane Battenberg

ASTIGMATISM

Astigmatism, according to optometrists, is the asymmetric shape of the cornea and/or lens of the eye, which causes blurriness in one area of an eye. It is like looking at your leg when you put it in water: the light refracts and makes the leg look off-center. The effect of astigmatism might be similar to looking through a glass with a wrinkle in one area; for that one area, the focus needs to be a little different to compensate for the distortion. In the eye, one may see farsighted or nearsighted in the warped area.

It is not entirely certain what physiological condition causes astigmatism. The cornea, lens or even the eye itself may not be rotationally symmetrical. Some people think the extraocular muscles are the cause for the deformity. Astigmatism may also result from a twisted spine, pelvis or neck as well as a tight or restricted posture.

The person with astigmatism can see things one way and then shift their focus slightly, causing things to look different. This can mean that they can see many different points of view with ease, but have trouble making up their mind as to which view they wish to adopt. They have trouble seeing which way things really are, as they keep shifting. Because the person can see things in so many ways, it is hard to make a decision.

In many ways, people with astigmatism are very consistent, yet there may be one area of their lives that seems inconsistent with the rest. Somebody could be very orderly in the way their house is laid out or the way they work, yet their garage is a complete mess, completely at odds with the rest of their house and personality. As another example, a person may have a healthy diet, yet when it comes to ice cream, forget it! It all goes out the window.

There could be a push/pull between how they are told life is and how they experience it. Their parents could have been inconsistent, pulling in different directions. There may be a conflict between what the person has been taught and their own thoughts or feelings;

thus they can see many different viewpoints, but have trouble seeing clearly which path to take.

The area of astigmatism in your eye is measured by an astigmatism axis and degree number by an eye doctor. If you imagine your eye like a clock, the astigmatism or blurriness can occur in different areas, like 12 o'clock (axis 180), 3 and 9 o'clock (axis 90), 2 o'clock in the right eye or 10 o'clock in the left eye (axis 045), or 2 o'clock in the left eye and 10 o'clock in the right eye (axis 045). (Your eye doctor can give you your axis).

Taking the idea that the mind affects how we see reality, the mind can blur or shut off sight in one area of a person's vision, which is what is happening functionally with astigmatism. The state of the mind's eye will affect the vision through one's fears, feelings, emotions and beliefs. Over time, this can affect the structure of the eye, actually causing physical changes in the shape of the cornea or lens. Having a physical change in the eye just means that the struggle with a particular part of one's reality has been there for a long time in their life (*Conscious Seeing*, Kaplan, p. 212). Even with corrective glasses, the "inner mind," where the source of the blur resides, is not illuminated. To fully explore the eye-brain connection, self-exploration can reveal and dissipate obscurities and distortions from the past that have blocked clear sight.

When life gives us problems, we may choose to shut down vision in one area in order to cope with the situation. According to optometrist Kaplan, each area of astigmatism has its own personality characteristics (*Conscious Seeing*, p. 213):

- 12 o'clock, the most common area, represents stubbornness, impatience and inflexibility.

- 3 o'clock and 9 o'clock represent a lack of commitment, not voicing one's truth and lack of love.

- 2 o'clock in the right eye and 10 o'clock in the left eye represent unresolved anger and resentment.

- 2 o'clock in the left eye and 10 o'clock in the right eye reflect an overly strong or weak will and sexual issues.

From an NLP standpoint, 12 o'clock, 2 and 10 are in the visual area, while 3 and 9 are in the auditory areas. Just knowing that astigmatism has a link with unresolved issues and emotions can help one get in touch with them. Allowing these emotions to bubble to the surface will provide the opportunity to see them in a new light.

CHAPTER 17

FACTORS AFFECTING VISION

EXERCISE, BODY YOGA

Part of seeing well is a process of knowing where we are in space and in relationship to everything around us. For this reason, exercise should be an integral part of vision improvement regimes. Taking walks or riding a bike engages the eyes to look at different distances, particularly afar and peripherally. There are moving targets to watch. Actively moving your body in these activities is better than passively watching moving targets, like being a passenger on a bus or in a car. It engages the whole body and brain, not just the eyes, waking up the ambient visual system and stimulating peripheral motion detectors in the retina (Orfield, p. 126).

Sports such as tennis and racquetball are excellent activities to help nearsightedness, as they engage and relax the eye accommodation. Body yoga, hiking, biking, posture training, dancing, movement, cross-crawling and even exercise on a mini-trampoline are all good ways to stimulate better vision. Being out in nature is a great way to both stimulate the vision and soothe the eyes. Taking frequent walks seems to help many of Orfield's nearsighted patients, who report improved vision as a result (p. 126).

When doing close work, take frequent breaks to rotate your head and neck all around. Relax your facial muscles, as they tend to tighten into a grimace and strain with concentration. Make sure to stop and look in the distance often to focus on faraway objects and close your eyes for a mini break. Do a few minutes of palming. Take deep, slow breaths to relax and to get more oxygen to the eyes. Blink frequently to keep the eyes moist.

Cross Crawling: This important exercise integrates both sides of the eyes and the brain. It is usually done standing up.

- Raise your left knee and touch it with your right palm.

- Then raise your right knee and touch it with your left palm.

- Continue striding (marching, swinging), moving forward, backward or in place, for 1–3 minutes.

- Keep your breath deep and easy as you enjoy the movement.

- A variation is doing this to rhythmic music.

This is a good exercise for sports. It is specifically recommended for skiing and snowboarding.

Have you ever mixed up two words, like "froove meely" instead of "move freely?" Or " breen groccoli" for "green broccoli?" A kid once told me that just meant he was "lysdexic!" This exercise brings the "cross-wiring" back into alignment.

Dr. Sam Berne, optometrist, lists common visual skills that involve vision as a more holistic process. One is bilateral integration, the lack of which produces word, letter and directional reversals, for which dyslexia is a catch-all term. Dyslexia means confusion and a lack of coordination and communication between both sides of the body, both eyes and both sides of the brain. Another skill needed for vision is eye-hand-body coordination, as in catching a ball, copying from the blackboard and drawing. Berne emphasizes the importance of vision and motor systems working together in a flexible, integrated way. He says that if anyone has had learning difficulties in school or coordination problems in sports, it may have nothing to do with their intelligence but may be due to inefficient vision. He correlates the specific types of exercises and the related visual/body skills that can be improved in his book, *Creating Your Personal Vision: A Mind-Body Guide for Better Eyesight* (p. 79). The different activities build on each other:

Practice Area	Improvement
Peripheral Vision	Movement/Balance
Visual Focus	Concentration
Eye Movement Control	Tracking as you read
Visualization, Visual Memory	Learning, following directions
Bilateral Integration	Overcoming dyslexic patterns
Hand-eye Coordination	Sports, Handwriting

Whatever physical activities you do, get the feeling of being centered within yourself as you use your visual awareness of where you are in space, balancing and centering inner feelings and emotions that may be stored in the musculature of the body. The more you can balance inner feelings with centeredness in the physical body, the better control you have over external forces. For astigmatism, the connection between one's body awareness and one's location in space relates to vision; inner calm is important.

POSTURAL TRAINING

Since vision is a motor act, exercise and posture have an influence on the health of our vision. Just for grins, try this simple test. Raise your chin and tilt the top of your head back. Notice if this makes your vision blurrier. Tipping your chin down should also produce a blurrier view. Now straighten your head and spine and look ahead. Did you notice your vision becoming clearer upon completion of this exercise? You can improve your distance vision by straightening your neck, moving it up and back. This demonstrates the way in which good posture relates to good vision. There are a number of techniques that may prove helpful in improving posture, one of these being the Alexander Technique.

Originally developed for people in the performing arts, it quickly gained a wider usage for anyone with muscular strain. It is a system of mind/body awareness with particular emphasis on the head, neck and back and their relationship to the posture and health of the whole person. Alexander teachers often noticed that their students' vision improved. It is frequently combined with the Bates Method to augment results.

If you are required to sit for long periods of time at a computer or desk, use a pillow for support in the small of your back. This arches the back and neck into a more natural curvature while relaxing the body. Keep noticing if your spine is comfortably erect or distorted. Take frequent rests to just look away (changing the distance range of your focus). Close your eyes or stretch your arms above your head to break the repetitive, habitual stance of the work.

Astigmatism may result from a twisting of the neck, spine or pelvis. People with astigmatism often have tight or restricted movement and posture. Paul Harris, behavioral optometrist, found that posture and astigmatism may be linked when one's body is habitually not aligned vertically. He found astigmatism in concert violinists, who habitually turn their heads in the direction of the violin (Kaplan, *Conscious Seeing*, p. 227). It is very important to maintain straight head and spine alignment, especially in a job that requires repetitive motion, or while reading, working at a computer, doing desk work or reading in bed with the book to one side.

NUTRITION

The eyes and the brain represent 2% of our body weight, yet they require 25% of our nutritional intake. Our eyes can use one-third as much oxygen as our heart. They use more zinc than any other body organ, and they have 70% of the body's sense receptors. They are the entry point for 90% of all information we learn in our life. Out of 3 billion messages sent to the brain every second, 2 billion are from our eyes. (Blind people use other senses to compensate).

—Excerpts taken from Jacob Liberman's book,
Take Off Your Glasses and See

Nutrition needs to be taken into account as a factor in good vision. While this section is not a comprehensive review of the subject, some interesting highlights are presented here as "food for thought." Eating excessive amounts of sugars and simple carbohydrates depletes the body's calcium and the trace mineral chromium. These are needed for elasticity of the eye tissues and focusing facility. Ben Lane, New Jersey optometrist, found that the eye focusing system could go into a nearsighted spasm if the person ate too much sugar and simple carbohydrates. Kaplan (*The Art of Seeing,* p. 44) encourages people to avoid heavily fried and/or refined foods and to also refrain from overeating. He says the eyes are a dumping ground for toxic buildup from the liver and kidneys when they are not filtering the blood properly.

Medical doctors Rose and Rose write extensively about nutrition's link to good eyesight and discuss how to improve various eye conditions in their book, *Save Your Sight! Natural Ways to Prevent and Reverse Macular Degeneration.* They give specific vitamin and mineral recommendations in addition to antioxidants. They also recommend reducing stress because of the chemicals that stress releases, such as cortisol, which weaken muscles and diminish the ability of antioxidants to nourish and protect eyes. They cite substances that are known to be toxic to eye nerve cells, such as cigarette smoke, MSG (monosodium glutamate) and aspartame (Nutrasweet, Equal). Both MSG and aspartame contain exitoxins, natural amino acids that can over-stimulate brain cells to their detriment. Side effects include memory loss, foggy thinking and dry eyes.

Emanuel Josephson, a New York opthalmologist, linked myopia to a lack of salts in the body fluids, due to a malfunctioning of the adrenal cortex. He found a diet high in carbohydrates, starches and sugars and low in proteins and fats correlates with developing nearsightedness, probably as a result of vitamin deficiencies. P. A. Gardiner, a London ophthalmologist, also found a link with poor nutrition. He found that myopic children were more likely to shun animal protein foods. This link to protein in the diet also showed up in another study of Eskimos by Elizabeth Cass. Myopia was unknown in the parents, but children, after changing from a traditional high protein diet to a diet of "white man's food" high in carbohydrates, became nearsighted (Eulenberg, p. 9).

Prolonged seeing at a close range may affect the blood circulation and oxygen to the eyes because a large amount of nerve energy is used by the visual centers. Oxygen is used up in this process when it not only goes to the eyes, but feeds the brain. Good nutrition depends in part on a healthy nervous system. Doing too much visual close work exhausts the nervous system, affecting the blood supply not only to the eyes but the whole body, including the digestion system (Eulenberg, p. 10). It is suggested that when you are doing close up work, make sure that you are breathing deeply and regularly. Intense concentration tends to constrict the breathing, while deep, slow breaths relax the body.

STRONG LENS PRESCRIPTIONS

If at all possible, it is better to wear glasses intermittently rather than all the time. Wearing glasses never improves the eyes. It only allows the eyes to see more clearly while they are worn. Many people have been told that if they do not wear their glasses, their eyesight won't improve or will deteriorate. Actually, removing your glasses (lenses) and learning to use the glasses only when necessary is the first step toward improving your vision. Basically, your eyesight fluctuates. It is not consistent from one moment to the next. Glasses, however, lock the vision into a set mode of correction, which does not allow the eyes to fluctuate, even though it is normal for vision to change. If, for example, you do Eye Yoga exercises and wear your lenses less frequently and your eyesight improves, your glasses won't automatically adjust themselves to that improvement.

We spend most of our time shifting our vision between various distances. We may not need lenses except for particular short-term activities, such as driving, night driving, watching performances or sporting events, reading, computer work, and maybe watching TV. Because of the shifting distances, we have some options. We can see with less than full acuity and tolerate a little blur, unless there is a special need for lenses as mentioned above. Learning to live with a little blur encourages the eyes to overcome or lessen that blur, whereas lens corrections have the opposite effect of worsening eyesight.

Wearing glasses and contacts usually worsens a person's unaided eyesight. Reportedly in Russia during World War II, many young men who didn't want to be conscripted into the military would wear strong glasses for several days before their eye examinations so they would fail and be rejected. Since lenses interfere with light transmission, color is not as intense with them, thus interfering with the perception of forms. Besides all this, wearing glasses, particularly for a progressively nearsighted person, can quickly become very addictive (Gallop, p. 116).

Nearsightedness lenses that are stronger than necessary tend to fatigue the eyes. These prescriptions actually produce stress and muscular tension. You would probably most notice this the first few days of wearing stronger lenses. Strong lenses also shrink internal levels of flexibility and sensitivity because the lenses distort size and distance. They can cause a person to withdraw even more from the external world, since the world is not seen as it really is. For many people, this often leads to a tendency toward being less flexible in their thinking and feeling, as well as problem-solving and decision-making.

According to Gallop (p. 116), once a person begins to use lens correction, their condition moves from one that is possibly transient to one that is permanent and likely to deteriorate over time. Strong lenses may, in some cases, even *cause* tissue changes in the eyes, increasing myopia. Dr. John Thomas (Orfield, p. 130) speculated years ago that the retina exerts a control on eye growth by releasing regulatory molecules whose production is influenced by the pattern of light stimulation.

Getting free from dependence on excessive visual acuity can allow the person the flexibility to restore their natural acuity. Some optometrists work with patients to improve their vision by getting them used to progressively weaker glasses. This reverses the process of adapting to stronger glasses and to a progressively more warped space world. The lens prescription then becomes a tool instead of a crutch.

HEREDITARY FACTORS

Hereditary factors affect us all in some ways. One can definitely see family trends in vision traits. Knowing our parents' ways of seeing could reflect our own perspectives and ways of thinking and give us a little more choice. Kaplan says that some researchers estimate 10 percent of the population is born with "congenital carryover," but there's a big discrepancy between that and the 55 percent of our population that now needs glasses. During the critical growing-up time, up to around age sixteen, critical events occur that may trigger the latent genetic factor (*East West Magazine*, p. 43).

The theory that nearsightedness is hereditary would get us off the hook, allowing us to point the finger at our genes, but it hints at general tendencies that aren't enough to make the case conclusive. Eskimo parents and grandparents who had lived a traditional Eskimo life had almost no nearsightedness (less than 2%). However, 58% of their children, who had all gone to school, were myopic, with the severity increasing with the number of years in school (Eulenberg, p. 5). Whether and to what degree eyesight conditions are actually hereditary is still being debated.

VISUAL IMAGERY

Visual imagery is widely used in a variety of ways. For example, it is used by athletes for motor rehearsal to improve their skill and performance. Many studies have shown mental rehearsal to be as effective as actual physical practice in improving athletic skills and performance in competition. A well-known basketball study had one group actually practice making successful free throw shots, another group *imagined* practicing making successful shots and a third group did not practice or imagine making shots at all. The improvement results were as follows:

Actually Shot – 24% improvement

Imagined Shot – 23% improvement

No Practice – 0% improvement

The imagined shots were most effective if participants also imagined the *feeling* of making the shots. Visualization is a kind of rehearsal beforehand, and in some cases our actual survival may depend on it.

Thinking something can make it so. Alvaro Pascual-Leone, M.D., Ph.D., demonstrated this in a study where he showed similar brain map and muscular motor signal changes occurred between two groups practicing keyboard piano. One group physically practiced the keyboard while the other only practiced mentally. Although the mentally-practicing group's performance wasn't initially as great as the other group, it took only a single two-hour physical practice for them to equal the physical group's performance.

Visualization is used to improve image memory, which also opens avenues of creativity from the right hemispheres of the brain. As visual memory improves, less effort and time are needed to take in a concept or event. Words are bits taken in one at a time, whereas a whole scene can be visually absorbed all at once. "Eidetic imagining" is the ability to see a complicated picture by closing the eyes and recreating it in one's mind, right down to the last detail. Our perception, our art, and the way in which we express ourselves are all based on our way of seeing.

Visualization can also be used for relaxation or healing. One technique is to visualize a white light over your head and then focus the light on an area of tension or injury in your body. (This is an adaptation of a Rosicrucian imagery technique). Imagery can also be used successfully as an adjunct treatment for physical illnesses, such as cancer. O. Carl Simonton and his wife assisted many cancer remissions in this way, as described in their fascinating book, *Getting Well Again*.

One of our clients successfully recovered from a serious accident by including visualization in his therapy.

> "In the summer of 2005, I was a healthy and happy Ironman triathlete in training for my next event. While on a training ride, I was hit almost head on by a car that turned left in front of me. I suffered multiple injuries to my ribs, hands, arms, legs and the most severe one to my now shattered and crushed hip. The doctors said that I needed emergency surgery to repair my hip and internal bleeding. On the bright side, they said that my other injuries would heal and that I was lucky not to have hit my head. When I came into the hospital, I told them that I was an Ironman and that I wanted to be an Ironman when I came out. They looked skeptical but said that they would do their best.

> "The most devastating injury of all came when I woke up from surgery. The doctors told me that they were not able to repair the damage and had to totally rebuild the joint using a graft from my

pelvis…and…that my athletic career was likely over or at best significantly diminished. I had not injured my head, but my mind was broken.

"The doctors explained that I could not put any weight on the hip for three months. I spent a month in bed, a month in a wheel-chair and a month on crutches. During the downtime I had a lot of time to think. I really came to appreciate what a privilege it was to be healthy and I missed it terribly. I got tons of support from my training buddies and even got a signed "get well" poster from Lance Armstrong. All of the support was awesome, but I was having great difficulty getting my mind focused on recovery instead of the loss of my athletic lifestyle.

"About two months into my recovery and very frustrated with my helplessness to do anything but rest, I saw Jane. She explained to me that the mind and body were inseparable and that I needed to get my head straight in order for my body to heal. We worked on guided visualization techniques where I imagined energy flowing into my body and working to repair my injuries. Finally I had something constructive to do. In addition to scheduled visualization work, I used the techniques to quash intermittent feelings of helplessness and sadness. I stopped feeling sorry for myself and worked the techniques to align my mind and body in the single pursuit of overall healthiness.

"Thanks to Jane, I had the necessary tools to combine with my eventual physical therapy to get on and stay on the road to recovery. After three months, with mind and body in synch, my surgeon gave me the OK to get back on my bike, and I took the first pedal strokes toward my dream of making it all the way back. At first I struggled just to get on and off the bike and then to take my first painful shuffles trying to jog. The journey back has been full of super highs and super lows, but thanks to Jane, I had the tools to deal with them. Two years from the date of the accident, with lots of mind and body work, I was in the water at Ironman

Lake Placid ready to start the race. I set a personal best time that day and have gone on to finish two more Ironman events (with more to come). The doctors have said that my recovery is not a miracle, but is the kind of recovery that they would only hope for and would never promise. I am convinced that I would not have been able to accomplish this without the tools I learned from Jane. I now use the techniques in my daily life to keep my head straight and in alignment with the various challenges we all face. Thank you, Jane!"

—Bond Jones, Austin, TX

To try visualization yourself, imagine that your body is very heavy and your feet are deeply rooted into the center of the earth. Then get a strong friend (or two) to try to lift you. Next, imagine yourself light and airy as a feather, floating like a balloon and ask the friend(s) to try again. Did they notice any differences?

"Numerous studies have confirmed the fact that vividly experienced imagery, imagery that is both seen and felt, can substantially affect brain waves, blood flow, heart rate, skin temperature, gastric secretions, and immune response—in fact the total physiology."

—Dr. Jean Houston, *The Possible Human* (p. 11)

Dr. Jean Houston has developed a series of exercises with the "imaginal body" to contact the wisdom of the body through visualization and imagery. The imaginal body is the body image we have when we are imagining doing something, the body of the muscular imagination. By developing this imaginal body, one's mind and body are being integrated in a way that gives greater freedom and facility of movement, greater stamina, pleasure, strength and ease. When exercises are done to increase awareness of this imaginal, kinesthetic sense, and when this is joined with verbal suggestion, one can increase health, longevity and healing. Here is one example of Dr. Houston's kinesthetic body exercise.

- Step (or jump) forward with your right foot.

- Step (jump) back.

- Step (jump) forward with your left foot.

- Step (jump) back.

- Imagine stepping (jumping) *forward* with your *right foot,* while you actually step (jump) forward with your left foot.

- Imagine stepping (jumping) *back* with your *right foot,* while you actually step (jump) back with your left foot.

- Imagine stepping (jumping) *forward* with your *left foot,* while you step (jump) forward with your right foot.

- Imagine stepping (jumping) *back* with your *left foot,* while you actually step (jump) back with your right foot.

- Continue stepping (jumping) forward and back with each foot, engaging both your actual and your imaginal bodies in each step for a number of times.

- At the end, stand still and notice how you feel.

You can vary this by raising one real arm while imagining raising the opposite, imaginal arm; then lowering the real arm while lowering the opposite, imaginal arm. Then raise the real arm as you lower the imaginal arm; raise the imaginal arm as you lower the real arm. You can feel the mid-point where the arms pass each other. You can also lunge to one side, as a fencer would do, arms out in an "en garde" position, while your imaginal body lunges to the other side.

"It is our tunnel vision and singular sense of identity that often limits our sense of our own possibilities—and yet it is the genius of humans to imagine being something we are not, and thus to extend what we indeed are."

—Dr. Jean Houston, *The Possible Human* (p. 21)

Many optometrists and vision educators have used visualization successfully to improve their clients' eyesight. The techniques range from relaxation, awareness of what one's eyes are doing, "seeing far or near," to improving the imagination. We can all visualize by just making things up. To improve your mental imagery, practice to get more and more detail, both by remembering something you've seen and by constructing an image. These and other techniques not only help eyesight, but they improve memory as well. If a letter on the eye chart were blurry, Bates would have his patients *imagine* it being very close. This trained the brain to see clearly. In *Eye Yoga*, we recommend telling the eyes to sharpen up and see while imagining for just an instant that you can clear your vision. With practice, you can extend that clarity to longer periods of time.

On a final note, we would like to share the experience of our first vision improvement teacher, Suzan Wilkerson Dallé. She had been medically declared deaf but she could communicate with her class so well you would forget she couldn't hear. She was reading our lips, you might think. Yet after she had met you and picked up your vibration she could talk to you on the phone very well. I just couldn't believe she was hearing without hearing sound. So one day as we were leaving class and she had her back to me, I *thought* a question to her. "Suzan, what restaurant are we going to?" She turned around and answered me, giving me chill bumps all over.

Suzan had learned to circumvent the hearing loss with some other function. She explained that when she found she could *visualize* sound, she realized it was all connected in the brain. She would tell her students that visualization is more than sight and we need to use all of the sensory modalities. When a student was talking about a mosque, her voiceprint formed a mosque in Suzan's mind. Suzan told us that vision is the main sense, that the eyes make the last decision about something. We screen out part of our vision so we can see what we need to see to fit our own self-image, matching what we know to be true. We each see things differently. Our perceptions— what we intake, like color and emotions, even how we intake, like the mechanical differences in our eyes—are different. We only perceive 50% of what we take in. Then when the light scatters in the eye, we intake even less. Suzan takes in a total sense of the communication, grounds it, then brings it back up and gives the person an insight about what they said in a way they may not have thought of before. She says we are all one, not separate, like drops of water in a glass of water.

In explaining the neuroplasticity of the brain, Doidge, in his book, *The Brain that Changes Itself*, talks about when we lose one sense, as in deafness, other senses become more acute and take over the lost function. Not only does the quantity of the brain's processing become more active, but the quality of other functions become more like the sense that was lost. For instance, peripheral vision in the deaf often increases, and their eyes act more like ears in sensing the periphery around them (Doidge, p. 295–6). In Suzan's case, her brain increased her visual-kinesthetic-intuitive senses to act as her ears.

STRESS

Developing vision limitations may stem from a person's response to stress or to a highly-charged emotional situation. When people develop physical visual limitations, there may be psychological or emotional parallels that could be linked to those conditions. Once you are aware of how the emotional stresses in the environment can create vision limitations on yourself and your loved ones, you may be able to change them. Easing the situational stresses can relieve the tension in the eyes and lead to improved vision.

"Not only does the sight become imperfect (due to strain), but also the memory, imagination, judgment and other mental faculties are temporarily lost..."

—William Bates (Quackenbush, p. 388,
Better Eyesight Magazine, December, 1925)

You may recall that we have mentioned earlier in the section on nearsightedness that Bates was convinced that mental strain created vision functional myopia. He claimed that it was caused by the effort one put forth, a largely unconscious effort, to see the details of unfamiliar objects at a distance, like a blackboard or an eye chart. Bates also said that any muscular activity such as squinting, hunching the shoulders or tensing the neck, and not just the activity of the eye muscles, contributes to myopia. He discovered how to bring the visual system back into balance, with the most important factor being relaxation of the mind.

Conversely, working on vision improvement can also help change a person's perspective, which can bring better coping skills with life's problems. Maintaining or improving your sight may lead to gaining some control over your environment.

Vision

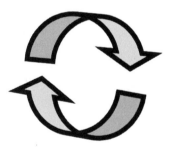

Life Stresses

As told in our Her-Stories section in the beginning of this book, Jane *improved her nearsighted vision* through eye exercises, thus gaining a much-needed bigger picture to deal with the many stresses bearing down on her. Martha *reduced the stresses* from a high-powered corporate career, which naturally resulted in seeing her life direction more clearly and an improvement in her distance vision.

Just as a better perspective on life can reduce stress and improve your vision, better eyesight can improve your perspectives on life.

CHAPTER 18

EFFECTS FROM VISUAL INTAKE OF LIGHT

Light taken in through the eyes can act like a nutrient to the brain, stimulating and waking up various physical, psychological and mental functions, such as increased field of vision, self-esteem and learning. The eyes are more than just relay mechanisms to the brain, like the skin when it relays sensory information. Since the eyes are hardwired directly into the brain, visual intake of light can actually affect the brain. Henning (1936, p. 10), as one of the pioneers in the use of light therapy, realized that vision is not a separate physiological entity in the body, but that it is intimately connected to the total person. Use of specific colors, rather than full-spectrum light, treated more than the symptoms of the visual system; it impacted the autonomic nervous system, which produced behavioral changes in his patients.

Colored lights have been used to improve a person's field of vision, which in turn has been closely linked with improvements in concentration, memory, attention span, reading and learning. A constricted field of vision and an enlarged size of blind spot have been linked to learning and reading problems. In the 1970s and '80s, optometric specialists began using Syntonic (colored light) therapy to expand the visual field. They used the visual field size to predict and evaluate functional visual problems affecting learning and general performance. While not one of the standard vision therapy procedures, it was successful in treating learning problems. General publications began reflecting growing research on the effects of light and color. For example, a *Southland News* article in 1982 entitled "Light Can Improve IQs of Children" reported that the mostly-red light from household bulbs causes people to make more mistakes, suppresses the brain's alpha wave rhythms and increases anxiety and stress. A July, 1982, *Reader's Digest* article stated that children's IQ tested 12 points higher in rooms painted light blue, yellow, yellow-green or orange. In black, brown or white rooms IQs dropped 14 points. That is as much as a 25-point difference depending on the color of the playroom!

In 1991 a *New York Times* article by Sandra Blakeslee reported that a team of prominent Harvard brain researchers had linked dyslexia to sluggishness in part of their visual system. The human visual system has two major pathways, the magnocellular, which sees motion, stereoscopic, depth perception, low contrast and objects in space, and the parvocellular, which carries out slower processes, specializing in color, detailed forms, high contrast and stationary images. Dyslexics have a slower magnocellular system. To read, the information from the magno system must precede the slower parvo system in just the right timing, otherwise words may blur, fuse or jump off the page. Evidence suggested dyslexia could be treated with colored light. Dr. Williams of the University of New Orleans experimented with colored light filters to improve the timing of the two pathways in dyslexia. She found that reading through blue filters helped 80% and red filters helped 8% of the children to read better (Blakeslee).

In addition to the areas of learning and the visual field, beneficial side effects of light therapy were repeatedly reported in the physiological and psychological arenas. In a study by R.M. Gerard in his 1958 doctoral dissertation at UCLA, adrenalin was activated and insulin inhibited by red light and vice versa with blue light. He found that colored lights have hormonal, sexual reproductive and activity-level effects on animals. Sorting through the many studies in this area,

Gerard found the emotional effects of colors on people vary. Physically, red was stimulating and blue calming. Thus a stressed person might view red as aggressive and anger-evoking, where a calmer person might find red stimulating and pleasant, bringing relief. The physiologically calming, slowing effect of blue might be psychologically arousing or depressing depending on the person.

The effects of light appear to influence the whole organism. Kaplan confirmed that children with reading difficulties also have reduced vision fields (1983). Colored light treatments made significant changes in their visual field as well as positive behavioral changes, while the vision therapy control group had no significant changes in either their visual field or their behavior. Liberman did a controlled study on the effects of colored light therapy on visual field size, memory, speed, and accuracy of eye movements with subjects with academic difficulties primarily in reading (*Journal of Optometric Vision Development*, "Light: Medicine of the Future,"1986). The experimental group viewed prescribed colored light frequencies four times a week for six weeks using a Lumatron machine. No other treatment or counseling was received by them or by the control group. Results showed the visual field increase for the experimental group was 208 times greater than the control group, their visual attention span was almost 4 times greater, their visual memory increase was 7 times greater and their auditory memory increase was 1.6 times greater.

The most revealing information came from parents and teachers in areas not measured, like handwriting, memory and emotional well-being improvements. Subjective changes included greater release of emotions, less hyperactivity, less tension and greater ability to handle criticism and confrontation. 75% reported improvements in their schoolwork, and the two who were on medication were able to totally eliminate their daily use of Ritalin. Withdrawn children came out of their shells, hyperactive ones calmed down and all became more open and emotionally receptive. Michael Hutchison in his book, *Megabrain*, concluded that the effects of the Lumatron can be "quite dramatic" and wide-ranging (p. 331–332).

Dr. John Downing, O.D., Ph.D., decided that it is light itself that programs our life energy rhythms, because photocurrent going from the eye to the hypothalamus sets the timing of the body's biological clock and thus the neural discharge rates of the hypothalamus. He combined traditional Syntonic treatment with a high optical quality light with a variable flicker rate, which entrained neurological rhythms during treatment. Using his neurophotonic device, the Lumatron, wavelengths of visible light pass through the eye, with the neural signals then passing through the retino-hypothalamic tract to the hypothalamus, and through the optic nerve to the limbic and cortical areas. Basically this increases the amount of electrical energy flowing into and throughout the brain, giving it more energy to do its work. He describes his technique as using the visual system as a direct sensory input to stimulate better brain function and balance brain/body chemistry. This enhances intellectual capacities as well as emotional and physical well-being. Just like taking vitamins for the body, it provides light as a nutrient to the brain. In his many case histories with children and adults he found his technique to be 95% successful in dealing with learning disorders. It is also highly effective in hyperactivity, headaches, fatigue and depression, according to psychotherapist Jill Ammon-Wexler, Ph.D. (p. 6).

In 1992, I did a study with the Lumatron to corroborate his results (Battenberg). The participants in my study watched a flickering, colored light for twenty to thirty-five 20-minute sessions. They completed a four-page profile at the beginning and the end of the series of treatments, noting any changes in physical, visual and perceptual, intellectual and emotional conditions. The profile categories were Stress Reduction, Visual Improvement, Attention/Concentration, Reading/Scholastic, Memory, and Emotional Stability. Pre– and post–field-of-vision tests were also administered to each subject. All participants effected an overall improvement in their visual field, which included: peripheral vision range in distinguishing movement and color, reduction in the area of their blind spot, and ability to distinguish a faster flicker rate before it fused to solid. While the sample size

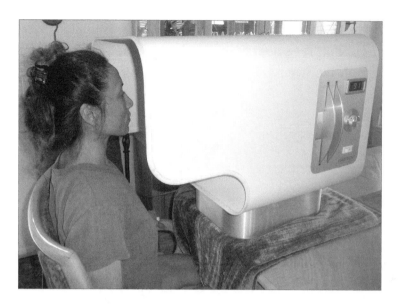

of my study was a limiting factor (fourteen participants), the results supported other research in showing the very powerful effects of light on a person's learning ability, visual field, and emotional and psychological factors.

The visual field results were as follows:

Blind Spot: (measured in millimeters)	Before	After	Average Reduction
	14.20	7.18	7.02

All subjects showed a reduction in their blind spot areas. The area of sight that could be expected to be recovered was the blind spot area outside of the optic nerve oval of 5.13 millimeters. The area was depicted by multiplying horizontal and vertical diameters.

Peripheral Color Distinction

Testing one eye at a time, subjects were asked to focus on a dot in the center of a page and name the color of the dot on a wand that was moved from the periphery toward the center. The wand was brought in at periodic angles so a roughly circular area could be drawn to show their peripheral field for each color. Everyone showed an improvement in each color and each eye except for one person, who showed a decrease in one color for one eye.

Average Gain (millimeters)

Green   15.34

Red   27.05

Blue   35.35

Peripheral Movement Distinction

Focusing on a center dot, subjects were to indicate by saying "now" when they saw a wand with a white dot approaching the center of the paper from the periphery. Again, the wand was brought in at different points to form a rough circle of their peripheral vision. All participants showed an improvement in their peripheral vision.

Average Gain (millimeters)

10–13 Sessions: 8.5

20 Sessions: 15.2

Incidentally, the improvement was greater than shown, as three people had peripheral vision beyond the edge of the test paper!

Critical Flicker Fusion

The efficiency of the eyes was measured by how long the subject could distinguish the flicker of colored light, using the Lumatron, as it was gradually increased from one to sixty flickers per second. The longer a person could distinguish the flicker, the more efficiently their eye was performing. Each eye was tested separately for both red and blue colors. All but one showed an improvement in eye efficiency, as measured by an increase in flicker rate before fusion.

Participants also noticed a corresponding change in from one to six of the categories in their profile. The improvements included the ability to intake and retain information, visual acuity, stress reduction, attention and concentration, and improved emotional states, as reported by the subjects. This measurement was a subjective rating before and after the treatments.

The number of categories that showed improvement was then tallied. Subjects reported changes in from one to six of the categories, as tallied below:

Number of Categories that Showed Improvement:

2 showed changes in 6 categories

4 showed changes in 5 categories

4 showed changes in 4 categories

1 showed changes in 3 categories

2 showed changes in 2 categories

1 showed changes in 1 category

Every participant reported some improvements. Participants that had 20 sessions (8) reported 77% of the categories improved. Participants with 10–13 sessions (6) reported only 53% of the categories improved. Other than expanded vision fields, the specific change patterns were unique to each person. Each had an exciting result to report, some of which are included below:

- The area I found the most improvement in was the intellectual area. My concentration improved a lot. I never fall asleep in class. Last semester I fell asleep about 75% of the time. This semester <u>one</u> time, only one! My reading ability improved, and I began reading more without problems. My memory seemed to improve because I would study about the same or a little more, but my grades improved a lot, from Ds and Cs to As and Bs. My attention span slowly improved as well. Thanks.

- Definite memory improvements and attention span. I haven't lost my keys for over six months, where I used to lose them all the time. School has become much easier, my short-term and long-term memory has improved astoundingly. No more cramming for tests, only a short review, then an easy A. Problems are handled with ease and minimal stress. Before if it didn't go my way I would freak out. I can attend four or more hours of school and still pay attention during that last few minutes. Before, 15 minutes was the most I could pay attention. I am generally more relaxed. I feel good about myself even though I am not working out daily. Before, I had to work out for hours every day to feel good about myself. In school I used to get Cs, now I only get As and Bs.

- I found myself wanting to read a lot more than I ever have. My colors have become easier to distinguish. I found that my attention span has increased on the level of letting my parents say what they need to. (This participant had only read a few books for pleasure in her life because reading was difficult. After the sessions, she went on to became an English major in college and later got her master's degree).

- I'm getting straight As (college)! I had a B in English, an F in Math, B in History and B in Psychology last semester. Now I'm getting straight As in all subjects, even though I'm not studying as much. When reading, I don't read some lines twice, like I used to.

- I can remember what I read better lately. I'm able to stay up later without getting tired. I'm able to concentrate (relatively unusual). I like this whole therapy a lot as I always feel relaxed when I leave. During finals I was able to pump out some papers in only a few hours and quickly complete a take-home final. My peripheral vision has greatly improved. While driving I feel more confident when changing lanes.

- (Eleven years old in Special Education): I feel like doing more exercise, like taking my dog for walks, playing catch and basketball, and I'm better with Nintendo. My reading and spelling are better. I was moved to a higher level in school and won a spelling award. I feel like seeing friends more often. (Note: When we first did his visual tests, his attention span was so short that it was difficult to get accurate results. We had to keep taking breaks and offering incentives just to get through it. During the final testing, his attention span was dramatically improved, and we only took one rest break).

- For a few days after a session I would feel calmer than usual. My back started to feel better and I wasn't as tired. I don't have to cover my eyes when I walk outside a classroom, as my eyes are much less sensitive to the light.

- I can go whole pages of a book without losing concentration, whereas before I couldn't even go a paragraph. Many times I felt a sense of peace and ease directly after the use of the machine. My emotional response to life improved tremendously. I now have more energy and feel much more happiness.

- The light machine seems to make my heartburn go away. I'm sleeping at night where before I just couldn't go to sleep! I take time off, go home and relax for myself, my mind says it's okay and the same amount of work gets done and gets done <u>better</u>. I guess I've lost a lot of my anger.

In addition to what the participants reported, their parents added insights of their own. Two said their sons had exhibited terrible temper tantrums, often destroying property, which disappeared after the Lumatron treatments. The participants seemed more mature, emotionally stable, able to focus on the task at hand and generally much easier to live with. This study supports other research showing the very powerful effect that light has on the whole person. Light, as a wave and a particle, is perceived by the brain as both energy and matter. It impacts all the master control glands and is significant in predicting the variety of changes that have been observed in this and other studies.

For over 100 years optometrists and healthcare professionals have been using colored lights as a form of treatment. The method of delivery has varied widely and been continually improved. With the Lumatron weighing around 70 pounds and not being readily available, it is fortunate that there are newer products on the market. The College of Syntonic Optometry has members who have developed their own light machines that are both portable and economical.

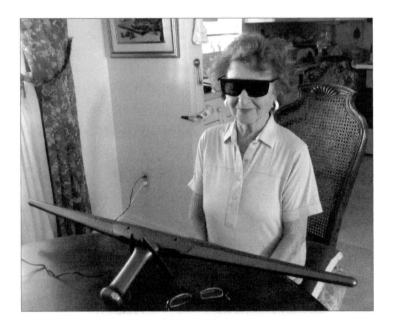

A relatively new technological breakthrough is the EYEPORT Vision Training System. It was developed by Dr. Jacob Liberman and has been cleared by the FDA. The EYEPORT utilizes red and blue lights to alternately stimulate and relax the eye's aiming and focusing system. This process retrains the eyes to function effortlessly, significantly improving aiming, tracking, focusing, teaming, depth perception, visual attention and overall performance. The EYEPORT has three programs, ten different speed settings and can be oriented horizontally, vertically, diagonally and from far to near, allowing you to train the eyes in different positions of gaze. It was found that EYEPORT makes a huge difference to learning-challenged individuals and those with ADHD, and has proven enormously helpful for pilots, computer users and athletes.

"I was able to make my eyes track objects better. My tennis game improved noticeably. I was able to track and see the ball better and hit the ball more consistently."

—Rich Allen, Irvine, CA

"After using the EYEPORT, I was in a state of dynamic relaxation, feeling more alert, relaxed, and engaged. I also noticed that things were easier to do and that both hemispheres of my brain felt in sync, as if I had done my brain gym exercises!"

—Martha Rigney

CHAPTER 19

VISION AS A METAPHOR

Many times the way in which people see is a metaphor for what else is going on in their lives or the way in which they are choosing to deal with situations. In this way, the physical manifestation or form of vision metaphorically reflects the structure of their situations.

When Nora first came to work on her vision, she spent a part of each session discussing the problems she was having with her husband. In one session, she became very upset, asking if it would ease the tension if she would get rid of all the furniture in the house because it was from her first marriage. Slowly, she began to see that she actually thought of *herself* as second hand. The problem was neither with her husband nor the furniture. It was how she saw herself that colored her world. The untruth exposed, she was able to see herself in all her beauty, wisdom and worth. All her "visions" improved (physical, self, marriage and life itself) and she saw her husband, herself and even the furniture anew. A happy ending for all.

Jean, an art teacher, was frustrated with her own paintings. She couldn't get all the details just right and was forever taking her glasses on and off. We worked with her eyes to change focus easily at different distances, at letting go of her view that it had to be perfect and moving into her own unique expression and creativity. She now reports tremendous freedom from lenses, no longer flipping her glasses on and off, and she is most satisfied with her artwork, feeling a freedom in its flow that she had not felt before.

One of a pair of twins came to our workshop. She was the good girl who always did what she was supposed to. She and her sister got glasses at the same time. Her sister refused to wear the glasses, broke them and kept losing them. She, however, wore her prescription faithfully, as she was told to do. When they became older, her sister was glasses-free while she wore thick-lensed glasses. Fortunately, she "saw the light" and was ready to free herself from her crutches with what she learned at the workshop. In her life and personality-wise, she was ready to explore life rather than just do as she was told.

Your eye condition may be trying to tell you how you are thinking. If you think of your situation in this way, you may gain new insights into the underlying causes. This may in turn lead you to consider ways in which you can shift your vision. Each person has their own internal reality and must decide for themselves what is true. Based on your own eye condition, use the chart on the next page to find suggestions for where to look for answers, ideas and new possibilities, in the event they resonate as true for you. The suggested affirmations can be used to focus your mind toward better vision. The New Sight column suggests new possibilities for seeing at a deeper level.

VISION CONDITION	METAPHOR
Nearsighted	Contraction. Fear of being overwhelmed by the big picture. Excessive attention to detail. Need to control. Critical, judgmental. Trying too hard. Withdrawal.
Farsighted	Keeping people and negative emotions at a distance. Need for space and independence. Focus on the future. Not "here-now."
Presbyopia	Getting old and fixed. Losing flexibility both physically and emotionally. Keeping emotions at a distance.
Astigmatism	Inconsistency. Mixed signals. Emotional confusion in some area of life. Tightness and restriction.
Floaters	Life is cluttered up with incomplete things floating around.
Glaucoma	Pressure building up inside. Unexpressed or unresolved dilemmas that build up.
Macular Degeneration	Giving up on life. Lack of motivation and purpose.
Retinal Detachment	Detaching from life. Losing touch with reality. Feeling abandoned by God. Unresolved grief or sadness.
Cataracts	Accumulations and clutter that cloud or impede flow, circulation and nutrition. Feeling stuck. Inflexibility. Uncertainty.

AFFIRMATION	NEW SIGHT
I look out at life with calm confidence and strength.	Seeing the world more as it really is at the deepest levels. Breaking down old boundaries of distinction and discreteness to create new syntheses, new cooperations, new possibilities.
I enjoy the pleasures of closeness, of focusing on the details and on my own insights.	Envisioning the whole, the largest picture. Global thinking, synthesizing parts into a cooperative, ecologically-beneficial whole.
I enjoy myself and my feelings. I am fluid, flexible and in the prime of my life.	Able to move easily between detail and big picture, micro and macro, emotions and abstract thought.
I continue to gain insights into old situations and perceptions to see new choices and possibilities.	Able to see all points of view in order to create harmony, clarity and consistency.
It feels good to clean out or let go of old influences from my past.	Able to separate the important from the unimportant. Able to focus on purpose and the more compelling issues without being mired in the mundane.
Each day I deservedly treat myself to moments of relaxation and play.	Able to find ways to handle the increasing pressures of our world. Conflict resolution. Cooperative efforts superseding competition.
I find new possibilities and enthusiasm as I refocus on my gifts and purpose.	Rediscover what's really important at a higher level of awareness, what life is about, greater context for being. Consciousness.
I am loved. I am an intimate, essential part of a larger family.	Reclaiming spirituality and connection with all. Interconnectedness of humanity and of all life.
I am impelled to clear away any blocks to my clarity.	Unclogging filters for life and letting the increased flow stimulate passion and enthusiasm. Taking in nutrition physically, emotionally, mentally and spiritually.

We are indebted to Roberto Kaplan and to Louise Hay for their charts on the body and mind connection in different conditions, which gave us the foundation for creating this one (see Kaplan, *The Power Behind your Eyes*, and Hay, *Heal your Body*).

HIERARCHY OF VISION

So far, we have focused on the physical, emotional and mental aspects of vision involving these faculties:

- objective seeing, perception
- focus, concentration, goal-driven intentions
- comprehension
- beliefs, what we "have eyes to see"

Little has been said about any visionary or spiritual aspects. If one views vision as a metaphor, the logical next step is toward the visionary or transcendent aspects of vision.

The vision faculties involved with these are:

- Imagination, creative visualization
- Conceptualization, manipulation of ideas
- Psychic abilities, clairvoyance, "second sight"
- Transcendental vision

These abilities evoke the transcendental and collective-mind dimensions; the place where what one envisions gets created or becomes a reality. Like a magnet shapes the iron filings on the paper above it, visions shape and form reality. There are cultures, specifically some Native American and African traditions, which use vision quests to initiate their youth into adulthood or to provide spiritual guidance in times of need. Great visions are also an important part of religions, world views and belief ideologies (the "isms": communism, capitalism, etc.). Corporations and nations use collective visions to gain allegiance and alignment. Visionaries, such as Martin Luther

King and Gandhi, held the pattern and the vision for changing the world. Increasing our ability to hold visionary patterns increases our effectiveness and power in the world.

In our society today, our collective vision is shaped to a large degree by the media. Whoever controls the media, controls our consensus reality, according to writer/astrologer Raye Robertson (p. 27). Her valid concern is that when we let an external media control our vision of reality (through television, printed news, computers, film, and so forth), we are actually giving up our ability to be self-reflective and to learn abstract thinking. In addition, she sees media as encroaching on our "bridge to Spirit" by supplying the visual images for us. This view is presented here to add one final layer as food for thought in the exploration of the concept that "how we see is how we think."

COMMON VISION MYTHS

There are some commonly accepted beliefs about our eyesight, myths that for many have turned into self-fulfilling prophecies. How many of these have you accepted as true?

☐ Vision inevitably gets worse as we grow older.

☐ Like a car, our eyes are mechanical and seeing is only a physical process.

☐ Once vision deteriorates, it cannot be recovered.

☐ 20/20 vision is necessary. It is the right goal for everyone.

☐ The shape of the eyeball stays the same and doesn't respond to environmental input.

☐ If you don't wear your glasses, you'll ruin your eyes.

☐ Too much close work will make your vision deteriorate.

☐ There's no relationship between vision and personality.

While many people have talked about these, we would like to acknowledge a few of our sources for the above "myth conceptions":

- Steve Gallop, "What's So Great About 20/20?"
- Lisette Scholl, *Visionetics*, p. 11–14.
- Martin Sussman, *The Program for Better Vision*, p. 11–15.

CHAPTER 20

FORM AND FUNCTION

How we use our eyes affects how we see.

—Jane Battenberg and Martha Rigney

The form of vision relates to the physical structure of the eye, such as the eyeball, the cornea and the lens. The function of vision relates to the way in which we see. Like the question, "Which came first, the chicken or the egg?", one might ask if function affects the form or structure of the eye or if the physical form affects the function.

Form: Does the form of the eye affect our mental and emotional thinking as well as our personality? Does blindness, color blindness, blurry vision, double vision, crossed eyes or wall-eyes affect our perspectives on life?

Function: When one overuses the eyes in close work, does this eventually cause the eyeball to change its form? Does a habitual, prolonged, emotional issue eventually contribute to a more permanent physical deterioration?

FORM FOLLOWS FUNCTION

When myopia gets worse, due to increased lens strength, much near work, habitual muscular tension or mental strain, it is called "functional myopia." It can eventually lead to a structural elongation of the eyeball, called "structural myopia." This is a case of form following function, where the habitual functioning eventually actually affects the form of the eyeball structure.

> "Myopia is a prime example of what is called function affecting structure. The more we read and do computer work and the more time we spend locked in tasks involving near vision, the more difficult it becomes to see at a distance. Book learning involves tightening the ciliary muscles to see near, and the longer these muscles are tightened, the more difficult it becomes to relax them when the task is completed. Further, this tightening of the ciliary muscles around the lens over time actually causes the eyeball to lengthen, creating an artificial but quite permanent myopic state."
>
> —Marc Grossman (p. 80)

One way that function can affect form is by wearing lenses more frequently or all the time, instead of only when needed. Increasing the strength of the prescription causes the eyes to adjust, making unaided sight even worse. Over time, frequency of wear and strength of correction can cause structural adjustments to the physical eyes.

> "When you were explaining how nearsightedness is related to the closing in of your world and becoming isolated, I began to feel very emotional. You were describing my life! At age seven I began to have trouble seeing the blackboard, so I was fitted with glasses. My Mom, wanting the best for me, encouraged me to wear them all the time, thinking that would be the best. As a result, I didn't play ball or other sports, I couldn't ride a bike and I spent all my time indoors, alone, reading. I felt isolated and

excluded from group activities of my peers. So I withdrew even more into the world of books. And of course, my eyesight continued to deteriorate, until today I wear lenses from the time I get up until I go to bed."

—D. L., Leamington Spa, England

Another way of increasing functional myopia (which can lead eventually to structural myopia), is to use the eyes in a repetitive habit, which over time causes a limitation. If you do close-up work all day, such as computer work, your eyes are seeing at a certain distance for many hours at a time. Over time, your eyes will adjust or "deteriorate" to become nearsighted.

> The way to change your vision is to change your habits of how you use your eyes. First become aware of how you are using them. Are you holding your breath or breathing shallowly? Do you tend to stare for long periods without blinking? Are you emotionally and visually pulling in or distancing?

Still another way that function creates a change in form is in response to stress, as we talked about above. For instance, a child who is afraid of a strict, commanding father might retreat into a shell, pulling his clear vision in as well.

Alice grew up in a home with an alcoholic father. She would escape his tirades by burying herself in a book or by daydreaming of being outside the house and in the clouds. When we explored her vision together, we found her vision was good very close and out in the distance, but it became blurry in the 2 to 15-foot range that we normally use in the house. She realized that emotionally (functionally), she protected herself in this "father in the house on a tirade" zone, and then structurally created her imperfect vision there. With this new awareness and insight, she was free to change her functioning, to use her many "adult" coping skills and let go of the form (myopia) that no longer served her.

When vision limitations are seen as symptoms of a larger problem, rather than the actual problems, you can get to the deeper issues. Your vision can indicate how you are responding to or dealing with life. Form follows function. If you are functioning emotionally or physically in a certain way, your physical structure will move into a form to accommodate that function.

FUNCTION FOLLOWS FORM

Form can also affect function, in that if you are color blind, lose sight in one eye or get cataracts, the limited structure will, of course, affect your functioning as well as your thinking. A color blind person notices shades and nuances of their monotone world as much as someone who sees all the color hues. In this sense, the limited color vision increased the person's ability to distinguish shades. However, the artistic beauty and joy of color isn't experienced in the same way as someone who can see all of the colors.

Our father lost most of the sight in his right eye as a young boy. That left him processing life in a right-brained way (left eye, right brain). He compensated by going into science, becoming a professor of statistics. Still, he wasn't completely analytical, often following hunches and intuitions. Although he had compensated for a physi-cal *form* limitation, his natural tendency to process in a right-brained way was evident, in particular via his global outlook, founding the Department of International Studies at his university and looking for global patterns at the local level.

Form

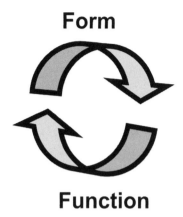

Function

The important factor to be aware of is that repetitive patterns, emotional stresses and physical limitations can have long-term effects on your eyesight. The converse is also true. How you function physically, psychologically and metaphorically is influenced by the structure and form of your eyes. Function and form are interrelated, and interconnected—as above, so below, as within, so without.

"How unseemly, how much less than fully human, to enter one's grave without having seen the truth of one's condition and without having ever taken one's condition in hand and changed it, radically adjusted it, of one's own volition and by one's own power, changing, for example, one's eyesight from poor to sharp, or, greater yet, one's way of seeing from deluded to illuminated! Both can of course be accomplished. The shape of the eyeball can be changed, as can the shape and entire functioning of the whole body. So can the perspective of the mind be changed."

—Joanna Rotté, Koji Yamamoto (p. 11)

The Media as the Form

In the '60s Marshall McLuhan coined the popular expression, "the medium is the message." McLuhan, Canadian educator, philosopher and communications theorist, proposed that the form of the medium molds our thinking much more than the content being delivered, by the very characteristics of the medium itself. The technologies used to deliver the message profoundly and insidiously shape the individuals and by extension the society and the culture. McLuhan warned that the electronic media was creating an overly intense, wired people with short attention spans.

Today the effects of watching TV from an early age can be tracked. Numerous studies show a correlation with increased restlessness and attention span difficulties. The fast pace and rapid shifts of the visual images require a speeded-up and perhaps more superficial visual processing. Then there is the addiction to computer/video games. The games trigger the release of the neurotransmitter dopamine, which is also released by addictive drugs. "People who are addicted to computer games show all the signs of other addictions: cravings when they stop, neglect of other activities, euphoria when on the computer, and a tendency to deny or minimize their actual involvement." (Doidge, p. 309)

Now add in the increase in text-messaging, the internet, iPhones and Blackberrys that are shaping and reshaping our brain patterns. These electronic media are powerfully effective at altering our nervous systems. In some cases, college professors are being forced to water down the difficulty of their courses to match the incoming students who are products of the new technologies. The brain has a plasticity that allows it to reorganize itself moment by moment. The *forms* of the media are subtly yet profoundly reshaping the *functions* of not only the individual but the very fabric of our culture and society.

Form and Function in Neuroplasticity of the Brain

First let's look at a person who has had a stroke. Their *functioning* will have been impaired by the change in the brain's *form*, the damaged part due to the stroke. By doing eye exercises, body exercises, speech therapy and other brain remapping exercises, a stroke victim can create new and rerouted neurological paths in their brain. Practicing *functions* literally changes the *form* of the brain's neuronal pathways. Recall the professor in Doidge's book who, after a stroke left massive damage around the brain stem, miraculously regained his abilities to walk, talk and write. He went on to return to teaching, hiking, biking, remarried and had a full, active life. When he finally died of a massive heart attack, the autopsy revealed that the damage from his stroke around the brain stem was still there. He had totally circumvented all that damage to become fully functioning and active.

Doing eye exercises (function) can change the brain (form), with its plastic qualities. Being aware of the vast potential of the human brain can inspire us to continue on the path of increasing our own neuroplasticity.

CLEARING BLOCKS TO VISION

CHAPTER 21

EMOTIONAL BLOCKS AND LIMITING DECISIONS

Dr. Jacob Liberman, author of *Take Off Your Glasses and See,* says, "Every time we express ourselves, we lose a little more emotional clutter." He links vision problems with resisted feelings and traumatic events, saying that it is much harder to see clearly when we are not expressing our feelings clearly. He has found in his work with clients that there has been some kind of major emotional stress one to two years prior to their vision first deteriorating.

Earlier we talked about emotional or mental stress being linked to deteriorating eyesight. In section 3 we discussed "how you see, is how you think" and "form follows function." In this section, we are going to take that a step further into the emotional and mental aspects. A person's mental/emotional state and beliefs can correlate with their eyesight. Our mental/emotional condition is often a result of patterning established long before we can consciously remember. By actively re-imaging some imagined or remembered past event to create a healthier, more generative state, we can influence our present state. This is because the unconscious mind cannot always distinguish between an imagined event and a real event. Given the choice, the unconscious mind will more often than not choose to follow the one that feels better and is less limiting.

The following is a simple process using Time Dimension Therapy that can be done with a partner by having them read the script. If you prefer, you may do the process alone by recording the script and playing it back for yourself. It is suggested that you read the script through once before reading it for a partner or recording it. This scripted exercise concludes the work done with a partner in section 2.

The process asks you to go back in time to when you first decided to limit your eyesight, where limiting your sight may have been used to resolve some dilemma. Bringing resources back to that time, you now encourage the earlier you to remake that limiting decision and envision better sight. In our Eye Yoga Workshops, many people report that their eyesight improves and they gain a new relationship with their eyes as a result of this process. Here are a couple of workshop participants' descriptions of their experiences.

"I went back to when I was turning fifty and going into a divorce. When we separated, overnight my eyesight deteriorated. I remember I was in Safeway grocery store and realized I couldn't see down the aisles! I was shocked to find that my distance vision had gone so suddenly. The Eye Yoga class pointed out the metaphor of being in Safeway and my vision of the future becoming blurry as the "safe way" to deal with things! I hadn't thought of that, but it makes total sense. My eyesight stabilized for some time after that until I got into a very emotionally bad relationship. Then my near sight began to get worse. This time I didn't want to examine the emotional, unhealthy entanglements, so I literally "shut an eye to it all." Now, after the Eye Yoga Workshop, I have a sense of insightfulness into the relationship between what's going on in my personal life and my eyesight. I can see that it metaphorically and literally enacts my life. Knowing this gives me a sense of control. To the extent that I take responsibility for my life and growth, I also have control over my vision. This is a "safer way" than shutting down my ability to see clearly. I am committed to working on my self and my vision with a renewed sense of being able to improve both of them over time."

—Michele V., Laguna Beach, CA

"To get to a time before I first limited my eyesight, I had to go back to "pre-existence," before I ever separated from the Divine. As soon as I experienced the initial embodiment and I separated from God, my sight became limited. So I went back to before I separated from God and abandoned the idea of separation as a fallacy. Realizing that I am never separated from God allowed me to drop fear and stress. It's hard to put into words, this absurdity of believing the illusion that we are separate in order to take on physical form. But it's a necessary illusion. This was so profound that it left me in a state of tears, wonderment and bliss for quite awhile after. Also, my eyesight improved greatly! Even today whenever I see problems as an illusion or a fallacy, just like being separated from the Divine, my vision clears. This is one of the most significant things about my vision, that when I get the big idea, even the ridiculous gets clear. This now applies to my everyday life, allowing me to see events in their reality rather than the dream they seem to be. And I love to see clearly!"

—Chavanna K., Costa Mesa, CA

TIME DIMENSION THERAPY

Partner's Job

Let's move on to the last exercise you will be doing with your partner. For this you may prefer some slow, gentle music or sounds of nature to be played in the background. Music without words is preferable, as words can be distracting. Read the following script in a slow, languid tone so that the very pace of your voice can lead the person down into a state of deep relaxation. The rule of thumb for reading this should be to "start slow and taper off." Please remember that the partner should read through the following script before reading it aloud, to familiarize themselves with the flow and sequence. The process should take 10–15 minutes.

Tell the person to get comfortable, usually with their eyes closed. Ask them to tell you what it is about their vision they would like to change or eliminate. For example, they may wish to improve their limited eyesight, correct their inability to see things close up or at a distance, or change the fact that it takes great effort to read in dim light. Then you will ask them if there are any emotions associated with the condition or the situation.

Script for the Process

Get comfortable, relax and close your eyes. …Relax your body, starting with your forehead. Let your scalp relax and let that relax-ation flow down into your face and jaw, letting them become very relaxed. Flow that relaxation down into all the muscles in your neck and relax your shoulders, letting them drop. Now let that relaxation go allllll the way down your arms to your elbows, relaxing them, and continuing down your arms to your hands, letting the thumbs and fingers and the palms of your hand relaaaaaaax. …Let all the muscles in your chest just go limp as a dishrag. Totally relax your diaphragm, your abdomen and your hips. Now let all the muscles in your back completely relax—just let them go. Only you can do this, only you can tell your body to relax. No one else can do this for you. Take control and relax all the muscles in your legs, your knees, and down to your ankles. Now feel your feet getting very comfortably relaxed. Relax the soles of your feet and your arches, even your toes.

For this you will be talking to your unconscious mind. There is no way to do this process consciously. Ask your unconscious mind, "Dear, sweet, unconscious mind, when did I first…decide…to limit my eyesight?" Just take whatever answer it gives you; don't think about it…When did you first decide to limit your eyesight?…If you were to know, was it before your birth…(pause), during your birth…(pause), or after your birth…(pause)? Before your birth, during your birth, or after your birth? Now, of course, you don't consciously remember before your birth, so make up an answer. Just notice the very first answer that pops into your head and take that one…[Note: Pause to let the person get a response. If you are the partner reading this script, you may ask them to raise their hand when they get an answer.]

If it was after your birth, ask your unconscious mind what age you were when you first decided to limit your eyesight?…If it was before your birth, ask if it was in the womb or before?…In the womb or before?…If it was in the womb, ask what month? Third month, fourth, fifth month? During what month did I decide to limit my eyesight?…If it was before being in the womb, ask if it was in a past life or ancestral, passed down to you as a family trait? If it was a past life, ask how many past lives back...Just get a number. You don't have to remember, you just want to make up an answer. So take the very first number that pops into your head…If it was ancestral, ask how many generations back the first time the decision to limit eyesight was made…Just raise your hand if you do not have a first event… [Note: If the person receives the information regarding the first event, then skip the next paragraph. If they have not found the first event yet, use the following script…]

Okay, you're going to just make it up. Ask your unconscious mind to recall the first time you decided to limit your eyesight…Was it in this lifetime or before…? Just make up an answer, choosing one or the other, this lifetime or before. Raise your hand if you did not get an answer. Just make it up, just choose one of those. If the decision to limit your eyesight was made before this lifetime, was it made in a past life or was it ancestral? If it was a past life, how many lifetimes back?…If it was ancestral, how many generations back?... Just make it up. If it was this lifetime, was the decision made in the womb, during your birth or after your birth? If it was in the womb, what month?... If it was after your birth, how old were you? Just get a number and take that. The first number that pops into your mind... Take whatever you think of first. Make it up. You don't have to remember consciously. [Note: Continue to ask these questions until the person comes up with a first event. Once they have received information about the first event, continue with the following section.]

Now that you have a first event, imagine that you can float above your life. Go ahead and float waaaaay up above your life, so that you see your life down below you like a river or a lifeline... It doesn't matter whether you see this lifeline or river or just sense that it is there. Good... Now imagine that you can take yourself back in time above that lifeline all the way back, whether it is straight or winding like a river. Follow it back until you are right above that first event... [Note: Pause here to give the person plenty of time to get there— around a minute or so.] Now look down at that first event and notice if it is night or day...Good...now, if it was a past life or ancestral, are you a man or woman, boy or girl?.. Look down at your feet and notice if you have anything on your feet. What are you wearing?... Do you get a sense that you are alone or with someone?... Are you alone or with someone?... If you are in the womb, ask if your mom is alone or with someone... And what are you feeling?... Notice how you are feeling and what is happening. This is the first event where you decided to limit your eyesight.

The unconscious mind may have limited your eyesight as a perceived "service" to you. It may have wanted to "protect" you so you wouldn't have to see, hear or feel some things that may have been too painful or difficult for you. But those things are in the past. It is important to learn from them and then let those old emotions and limiting beliefs go. Like peeling a postage stamp away from its paper, we are going to ask your unconscious mind to peel away those old emotions from the increased awareness and knowledge you have gained through this experience. Keep the awareness and knowledge that help you to do things better and drop those old emotions that no longer serve you. Like clothes that fit you in grade school, but that you have outgrown, they are no longer needed and don't fit. So keep the reframed new perspective and release the old emotions now.

I'm going to give you some time to explore what is happening at that very first event when you decided to limit your eyesight. Your job is to see *now* what the former you couldn't see *then*. You have many more resources now than you did before. Once you can see what you couldn't see previously, you will be able to help the person you were then make a different decision about your eyesight. So, gently explore the situation and act as a mentor or guide to your prior self. From this higher perspective, you can help yourself see the situation in a new light. It doesn't make anything bad that happened back then okay or right. You aren't condoning someone else's inexcusable behavior. You are simply getting the perspective you need in order to release any decision that limited your eyesight. Help the younger you see what they need to learn. [Note: Give 2–5 minutes or until the person indicates that they have finished.] Once you've helped the person you were back *then* to make a better decision about seeing clearly, indicate that by raising your hand. Notice the difference in how that person feels with the new insights. Feel that change in your body and in your emotions.

Very important note: Here are some instructions to follow in case the person drops into a very strong, undesirable emotion or memory. This almost never happens; however, you will want to be prepared in the unlikely event of an overwhelmingly strong emotion surfacing. Since you do not want the person to re-experience any traumatic event or emotion, you want to get them "above" that event. Tell them to come up out of the event and to look up with their eyes. Say something like, "*Look up, look up, look up and keep your eyes turned upward. Now go back, way back before that event ever happened.*" The key to this is to get the person's attention way above and prior to the event.

1. Keep the person's eyes looking up (into where the brain stores

the visual sense).

2. Get their attention focused on a time well before the emotions and the traumatic event ever happened. Ask them to go up as high and as far back as needed for this. From there, you can continue with the reframing and with getting the perspectives needed while reassuring them that they do not need to go down into the event to learn from it. Tell the person to sever all ties with that event. Say to them, "*The emotion doesn't protect you. What you **learn** protects you. It does not mean that what happened was justified or right. You are not condoning someone else's inexcusable behavior. You are just cutting the energetic links that have continued to feed that event so you can truly be free from it. You will no longer continue to give it your energy.*"

3. After saying this, have the person stand up and walk around, looking up if the traumatic emotion continues. It is important to continue the process until they can successfully access the time before the emotion and then come back to the present time. Continue the process or you run the risk of leaving the person in the traumatic emotions.

Once the person raises their hand, proceed with this part: Good! Congratulations! Now ask your unconscious mind if it is okay to keep this new awareness and higher perspective along with this new feeling to enable you to see better in the future. ... Great. Now come forward above your lifeline, fully aware of that new perspective. Feel the strength and wisdom that you have gained. Your job is to clear your entire lifeline of any restricting decision to limit your eyesight. Come all the way back to the present moment as if you have moved over a groove into a parallel reality in which you never decided to limit your eyesight. You are free of limitations in this reality. Notice how your life is *now* ... as you come all the way back to this present moment ... [Note: Allow several minutes, instructing the person to give a hand signal when they have returned to the present moment.]

I'm not going to suggest that **your eyesight will *improve greatly!***

You have the right to have eyesight as clear as you want to have. Now that you have returned to this present moment, gently float down into the room.…Comfortably come back into your body. When you are ready, open your eyes.…Welcome back. Take a moment to look around with soft, relaxed eyes and notice how things appear.… Has your eyesight changed at all? What has changed? Congratulate yourself on all the changes you have been able to make, no matter how big or small. An inside job usually creates changes outside, sooner or later.

What you have done is to establish a new bond with your unconscious mind. You are developing a rapport between your brain and your body. Maybe you can see more clearly. The quality of your eyesight is not as important as the relationship that you are cultivating with your brain, to be able to tell your eyes how and when to see. It is your unconscious mind that regulates all the autonomic functions in your body, so when you can talk to your unconscious mind, you can actually talk to your body. You can develop the ability to see clearly. Enjoy your new relationship with your unconscious mind. Enjoy the friendship you are developing between your brain and your eyesight!

Continued Use

If the emotions and decisions are still there and you would like to continue working with this process, you may go back and repeat the process until you are able to change your mind and let go of those old negative emotions and beliefs that no longer serve you. You may want to do it daily or weekly until you achieve the desired results. Any change, no matter how great or small, is a success because it means you can change your brain and change your sight. Congratulations!

More Client Experiences

- After doing the TDT process, I noticed that I could see a little clearer. But my glasses wouldn't work—they made things fuzzier. Then I realized that my prescription was too strong, so I started using an older, weaker pair.

—C. King, Orange County, CA

- It is hard for me to see near or far – everything is fuzzy and confusing. In this TDT process I realized that my poor eyesight started early in childhood. I was told that what I perceived (mostly about my parents' fighting) wasn't true. Since everything I saw and felt was invalidated, I found everything very confusing and fuzzy, and my eyesight followed.

—J. Waldram, Costa Mesa, CA

- A client with a detached retina realized that she had detached from life, as early as in the womb. When she said, "I was detached!" we both realized that it had become a metaphor for her eye condition.

- I did this TDT process in a workshop. While I did experience a slight improvement in my eyesight, the real value was deeper than that. It was just amazing what emerged from the process, and what an insight into myself it gave me!

—workshop participant, Guildford, England

From Color Blind to Full Color

"In school, I tested red-green color blind and even bright colors were difficult to distinguish: white from pink, blue from purple, red from green, yellow from lime green, etc. Rainbows were a disappointing 2 color smear of off yellow and blue. I looked for ways to correct this and the uncomfortable emotions I felt from being teased at home.

"The most dramatic improvement occurred in 1971 using an altered state meditation technique I discovered two years earlier. By consciously relaxing the muscles and defocusing my eyes, I learned to enhance awareness of depth perception and movement, variations of light and shadow, and had begun to see colors in auras around people and trees. One afternoon, filled with energy and an intense desire to see colors clearly, I went deep into an alpha state and focused the energy into my third eye.

"When I opened my eyes, I felt cool air penetrate my eyes. I was able to see and describe minute color variations with a friend. My eyes felt wide open, as if light bathed them with waves of color. For the rest of that day, my color rods revealed a wide spectrum of vibrant hues. The more I experimented with my consciousness of color and light, the more I healed my vision and emotions.

"Today I can identify colors, and I remember the startling clarity of those experiences. As my clients remove emotional blocks, they report that the room, the air, and colors seem brighter. I am committed to using techniques to improve color acuity. Reading your manuscript, *Eye Yoga,* reminds me of so much that matters. Thank you, Jane and Martha."

—Lance D. Ware, M.A., CHT

CHAPTER 22

BACKGROUND ON TIME DIMENSION THERAPY

HOW THE PROCESS WORKS TO CREATE CHANGE

The process used in the script to create change is a technique called Time Dimension Therapy (TDT). It came out of Neuro-Linguistic Programming and uses NLP techniques as well as a hypnotherapy visualization process. If you are interested in learning more about this process and about how change is possible, continue reading the rest of this chapter.

What is NLP?

NLP, or Neuro-Linguistic Programming, is a model of the *structure* and form of how our brain processes and makes our subjective experiences inside our head. It models how that determines our feelings and behavior. It is about the structure, not the *content*, of our subjective experiences.

It is a bit like watching ourselves think, learning how we "think ourselves into behaviors and states." In this sense, we are not looking at reality, but at the way in which we <u>experience</u> reality! NLP shows us how we construct our reality. Our construction of the world is like a map, which is only a representation of the actual territory.

When you first wake up in the morning, how do you remember who you are and where you are? How do you know what day it is, what things excite you or what your concerns are? You may say you just remember. Where is all that "memory" stored? How do you remember to have that same wrinkle or freckle when your skin cells are constantly dying, to be replaced with new cells? Is there some kind of programming or template that tells your body to keep reproducing itself in the same way it was, even though the cells keep changing?

You remember how to be "you" because you have memories stored in your mind/body via your five (at least) senses, as pictures or visual images, sounds or talking to yourself, feelings, sensations, tastes and smells. In NLP those are called your Internal Representations. They determine who you think you are, what you think is reality and the way in which you behave. In a sense, they act as the operating system of your brain (like a computer).

If, indeed, they are your operating system, then when you change your pictures and feelings of reality you are literally changing who you are. When you alter the internal representations of reality that you have, you are actually changing yourself—your beliefs, what you think is possible and not possible, how you feel, and even your physical body. The power to change lies in knowing how to get into those internal representations to change them for the better. "Change your mind and keep the change," as the title of an NLP book by Steve and Connirae Andreas suggests. We develop an internal neuropsychological representation of the world that forms the neuronal basis for all our habits, beliefs and overarching ideologies (*Brain and Culture* by Bruce Wexler, Yale psychiatrist and researcher). Michael Talbot, in his book *The Holographic Universe*, concludes the following after considering the theories of David Bohm and Karl Pribram. "Our brains mathematically construct objective reality by interpreting frequencies that are ultimately projections from another dimension, a deeper order of existence that is beyond both space and time: The brain is a hologram enfolded in a holographic universe." The brain converts waves and frequencies to make reality look concrete to us

(p. 54). Studies have shown that the visual information entering our brains is edited by our temporal lobes before being passed to the visual cortex. Some say less than 50% of what we see is actually from the information entering our eyes. The other 50% is formed from our expectations of what the world should look like (p. 163).

NLP Model of Reality: Let's look at a model of this to make more sense of it.

To follow this model, start with the arrows to your right. These depict external stimuli coming in at you. There are about two million bits of information per second that you could pay attention to if your neurology could take it in. Since this would overload your system with too much irrelevant information, the human brain sorts through the two million and takes in about 126 bits of information per second, according to Mihaly Csikszentmihalyi. "What determines which 126 bits are relevant enough to take in?" you might ask. The answer is your filters. They allow you to sort this information, so that you delete, distort and generalize the bits in order to organize them in a way that is meaningful to you. The information is displayed, stored and retrieved by your internal representations (your five senses) in pictures, sounds, physical and emotional feelings, tastes and smells. Your internal representations become the building blocks of your reality, determining your internal state and your physiology. Your behavior is a *result* of these two things. To complete the circle, your behavior determines to a large extent what then comes back at you from the external world—the way people treat you by how they respond to your behavior, and how your own beliefs shape your reality.

To review this process:

- An external event happens, and you become aware of it, taking it in.

- You run it through filters of your model of the world, such as:

  Your memories and life experiences

  Your beliefs, attitudes, and values

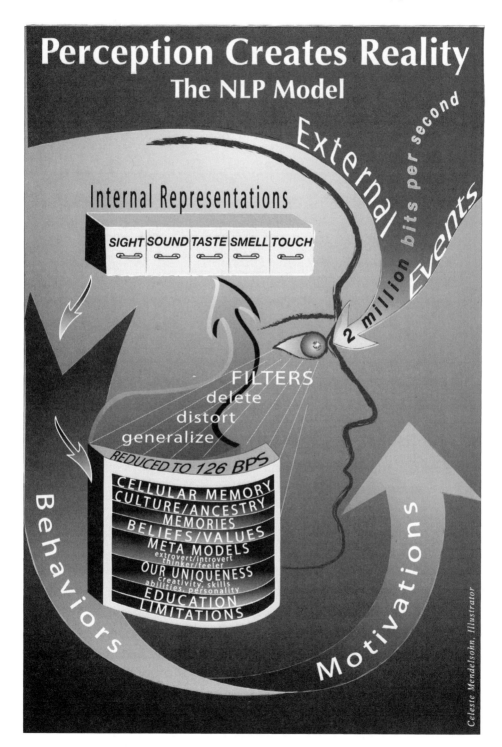

The language you speak

Time, space

Your meta-programs (introvert, extrovert, thinker, feeler, etc.)

- You delete, distort and generalize the input to distill it down, since you can only pay attention to a fraction of what comes at you.

According to Mihaly Csikszentmihalyi, we have a finite capacity to take in things. He says out of two million bits of data per second coming in at us, we can only take in 126. Imagine two million toothpicks floating by every second and you grab 126 of them to build your reality. What you grab, which bits you choose to pay attention to, is determined by your filters. You then build your internal representations, your internal reality, out of what you take in. You store these bits in pictures, sounds, feelings, tastes and smells, called your Internal Representations (*Flow*, p. 29).

- You make Internal Representations of the information, stored as pictures, sounds, feelings, tastes and smells.

- Your Internal Representations determine your physiology (body responses) and your state (feelings, emotions).

- Those in turn determine your behavior and reinforce or change your filters (beliefs, memories, attitudes, values, etc.).

- Your behavior and your beliefs, values, attitudes and life experiences shape to a large extent what comes back at you from the rest of the world. Not only does it influence how others treat you, but you interpret and make meaning of the external events based on what you expect, anticipate or believe. In this sense, you create your own reality.

The place where you can change your reality, where you can shift your own beliefs and have a shot at changing your physical body, your emotional reactions and what life gives you externally, is in the Internal Representations you make. Alter those Internal Representations and you are literally reaching into your brain to change its operating system, as in a computer. When you reframe your life experiences, when you change your memories of who you are, you change who you are, as if you are moving to a parallel reality or installing a new program or operating system in your reality. Remember, how you know to be who you are, is because you have these stored "memories" (Internal Representations).

In the movie, *The Family Man*, Nicolas Cage is taken back in time to how his life would have been if he had stayed with his first love in the small town they grew up in, working at a tire store for his father-in-law to support his wife and children. Then he is returned to his current life of a rich, cultured, single playboy on Wall Street. The perspective he gains from the visit to the past-that-could-have-been changes how he chooses to live differently in his current life.

Since memories change over time, they aren't *real* memories, but rather selective memories, like myths, that control your reality. When you change what happened in your imagination and rewrite your story, it is as if you flip over to another groove, a parallel reality. Imagine what your life would be like if you had taken a different road or made a different decision somewhere in life, like in the movie, *The Family Man*. Some say there are parallel realities of lives where we made different choices. When you go into a memory and reframe it, get a different perspective and learn from it, the change in perspective literally re-writes your history and who you've become.

In *Brain and Culture*, Wexler cautions that when we age, our brain neuroplasticity decreases. We ignore and belie information that is different from our internal reality. We tend to stay with the familiar, from our friends to our beliefs. We find it difficult to accept new ideas and perceptions. Gradually we shrink and micromanage our environment to make it comfortably familiar. Wexler's theme is that much of the global cross-cultural conflict today comes from a decrease in our brain plasticity or thinking flexibility (Doidge, p. 304–5).

We all have patterns in our lives made from our experiences, the limiting decisions we have made about ourselves or life, and the anger, sadness, fear and guilt from the past that we hold onto. It is as if we have a pattern for a shirt. It is out of style, frumpy and doesn't fit. No matter what kind of expensive, beautiful, tasteful, exotic new materials we may buy, we still get the same frumpy shirt from that pattern. In life, no matter which husband or wife, job or house you have, no matter where you move or what new relationships are formed, the same old patterns keep popping up. Like the shirt pattern, "Wherever you go, there you are!" It is only by changing the pattern that you can get a "new shirt" or change in your life.

Before going into ways in which we can change these patterns, there are a few more points that will help to set the stage for positive transformation. You might ask how changing something in your head can create changes in your body or the external world. There is a connection between your mind and your body that was first discovered in 1986 by Dr. Candace Pert. In her book, *Molecules of Emotion,* she writes of her groundbreaking research on neurotransmitters, and she provides scientific proof that the mind and body function together as an integrated system, linked by the neurotransmitters that form an information network between the two. Neurotransmitters can instantly change the body, since they are the communication link with every cell. Deepak Chopra popularized this notion by saying that your cells are eavesdropping on every thought you think (*Ageless Body, Timeless Mind,* p. 5). All of our thoughts turn into chemicals that travel throughout the body giving the message to every cell (*Perfect Health,* p. 109-110). Dr. Pert also reveals that all of our emotions are really chemical responses of hormones, peptides, opiates and other neurotransmitters.

Dr. Deepak Chopra says that our cells are eavesdropping on our every thought. Further, every cell has a "mind," its own intelligence, and creates messenger chemicals that are secreted in response to emotions, feelings and beliefs. This link between the entire body and what we feel happens instantly, at the same time.

The potential that the neurotransmitters have in our bodies is quite amazing. According to Dr. Paul Goodwin, University of Alaska, we have on the order of 100 billion neurons in the human brain, and each neuron ultimately connects to between 1,000 and 100,000 others, which makes 10,000 quadrillion potential neural connections (Goodwin, p. 18). That is a *lot* of zeros! In addition to the potential bioelectrical voltage impulses traveling these neural pathways, a host of neurochemicals establish a strong chemical communication between the brain, the body and even the mind (Goodwin, p. 31). The human cortex alone can make a million billion synaptic connections, with the number of possible neural circuits being ten followed by at least a million zeros, according to scientist George Edelman (Doidge, p. 294). These astronomical numbers describe the human brain as the most complex known object in the universe, capable of diverse mental functions from physical behaviors to various cultural activities and of continual massive microstructural changes. All this gives us a redundancy of at least three times what we need. According to Dr. Jean Houston, we use only 10% of our physical and 5% of our mental capacities. With so many potential neurological connections all activated by and responding to neurotransmitters, we are powerhouses beyond our conscious imagination.

A study that was done with a woman who had multiple personalities (MPD) represents a dramatic example of this power. She had adult diabetes, as confirmed by her blood work (BUN). In the experiment, she changed personalities, after which they immediately took her blood sample again. This time, the woman did not have diabetes. Instantly she went from having diabetes to not having it, only by changing personalities. That second personality did not have the same life experiences that had brought on the disease that the former one had. Another interesting phenomenon with some people with MPD is that their eye color changes with the different personalities that emerge. Some even have a drawer full of different strength glasses that match each personality.

Dr. Theresa Dale, naturopath, says: "When we resist an emotion and/or feeling, the resistance itself creates an electromagnetic charge of energy which stores on a cellular level in the organ or gland that correlates to the particular emotions. Over time, as the pattern of resistance continues, this charged energetic pattern creates more and more of a burden on the particular organ or gland where it is stored."

—Alexandra Delis-Abrams, Ph.D., "The Attitude Doc,"
Improved Health Through Honoring Our Feelings

Returning to the subject of the neuroplasticity of the brain, Eric Kandel, researcher from Yale and psychiatrist, has shown by brain maps taken before and after psychoanalysis that the therapy literally changed the patients' brains. By "talking to the neurons" we can alter their structure and strengthen the synaptic connections between them (Doidge, p. 133). Kandel was the first to show that our neurons change their shape and increase the number of synaptic connections with other neurons when we form long-term memories, for which he won the Nobel Prize in 2000. He showed that when we learn "...we can shape our genes, which in turn shape our brain's microscopic anatomy (Doidge, p. 220–1)."

Recent research and investigation by such people as David Bohm, Karl Pribram and Rupert Sheldrake, show that our bodies are, indeed, holographic in nature. Holographic means that every part contains a blueprint of the whole. When you shine a laser beam through a holographic photographic plate, you get a 3-D image, like R2-D2's projected images in Star Wars. If you were to tear that photographic plate into tiny pieces and shine a light through any of those pieces, you would still get the same 3-D image! Studies with salamanders showed that if you removed and minced up their brains and then reinserted even a tiny portion, they would still be able to function (Michael Talbot, *The Holographic Universe*). Just like the holographic film plate torn into tiny pieces, the salamanders were able to recreate the functions of the whole brain from a tiny piece.

Apparently in some cases people are able to function normally even without most of their cerebral cortex. In a 1960 article for *Science* titled "Is your Brain Really Necessary?" writer Roger Lewin quotes a British neurologist, Dr. John Lorber, who studied cases of hydrocephalus (water-on-the-brain). "There's a young student at (Sheffield) University who has an IQ of 126, has gained a first-class honors degree in mathematics, and is socially completely normal. And yet the boy has virtually no brain....When we did a brain scan on him, we saw that instead of the normal 4.5 centimeter thickness of brain tissue between the ventricles and the cortical surface, there was just a thin layer of mantle measuring a millimeter or so. His cranium is filled mainly with cerebrospinal fluid."

I first heard this story in a workshop, where a surgeon shared a similar story about his own father, a college professor. When his father passed away, he performed the autopsy on him and was astounded to find that his father had no brain except a few cells around the edge of the cerebrum. It was a mystery to the surgeon how his father could have functioned so intellectually. If these few brain cells around the mantle recreate the brain holographically, like in the studies with the salamanders, this opens up many new possibilities, not only for conditions like hydrocephalus and strokes, but for all of us. If we can recreate "lost" function, such as eyesight, this means we have tremendous capacity, far more than we may realize. We are not "mechanical," like a car. Rather, we are holographically, neurologically and neurotransmittally capable far beyond what is needed or expected as of yet. We have a huge capacity for change and experience that exceeds what we have thought was possible.

CHAPTER 23

THE PROCESS OF TIME DIMENSION THERAPY

When an emotionally significant event happens, we respond with a feeling or, perhaps, we make a decision. Later in life, some other event may occur that reminds our unconscious mind of that first event. The two events get linked in a gestalt, a stimulus-response. As life goes on, we have many of these gestalts that affect our behavior when they are activated. We usually no longer remember that first event, at least consciously; the stimulus-response pattern is automatic.

A client was afraid to travel by plane. When she did, she would have to lie in a darkened room for a day afterwards until the effects subsided. This was not useful, as she needed to fly as part of her job. When I would imitate the plane engine noise in an (RRRRR) sound, she would get a panicky feeling. I asked her when she felt that fear for the first time. She said when she was a little girl, a dog growled at her (GRRRRR). Later, a bee (ZZZZZ) stung her, and that hurt! Way out in the future, she developed a fear of planes.

She thought back before the first event when the dog had growled at her and there was no fear. She got the insights: the dog growled but didn't bite. Bee stings weren't really so scary even though they hurt. She released the fear from all those past events, linked by her unconscious mind to the sounds, back along her lifeline to now. Then, to test to see if the fear had completely disappeared, I repeated the (RRRRR) trigger once more and she didn't have a reaction. She flew home, and her doctor wrote me a letter saying she had no ill effects from the plane ride. Years later, she was still able to fly with no aftereffects.

Sometimes we make limiting decisions that affect us well into the future, like an unconscious programming. We no longer remember making the decision that formed the pattern, yet the pattern continues to operate.

A client came to me with a backache he had had his whole life. He could count on one hand the number of mornings he'd woken up without it. He'd had it checked out medically with an MRI and nothing showed. Massages didn't seem to help it. After some questioning, I asked him to talk to me about resentment—when was the first time he felt resentment? He said that was easy, when he was five years old, his Mother got sick and quit playing with him. He resented that she was no longer his playmate. I asked him what he decided, and he said, "I'd have to stiffen up and do it all myself!" I told him to go back and talk to that little boy and get him to make a different decision, and not to come back until he did! Pretty soon, he said the boy had agreed. He cleared that limiting decision all the way back to now, and his back didn't hurt. For the next several mornings, I received a phone call from him, amazed that his back still did not hurt. It's been over five years and that pain has never returned.

The process called Time Dimension Therapy involves the unconscious mind in a visualization process. It involves making up a scenario that you probably don't really remember, because it happened so long ago. Anyone can make up a story, so you will just invent a story. It's your own mind that is making it up, after all, so trust that "all roads lead to Rome," as the expression goes.

Let's talk a bit about the unconscious mind. You have a conscious, cognitive part of yourself, which we'll call your conscious mind. And then you have the part of your mind that makes your heart beat, regulates your chemistry and body heat, causes you to breathe automatically, and so on. That part of the mind, that you are largely unconscious of, is also in charge of such things as your memories, unresolved emotions, and most importantly your survival.

The conscious mind is very intellectual, while the unconscious mind is childlike. You may wonder why you need to concern your-self with the unconscious mind if it is not very sophisticated. Well, if you could have changed your patterns with your intellect alone, you probably would have done it already. The unconscious mind stores all of those old patterns that keep you doing the same things over and over again. It remembers all of those hurts, angers and fears, and all of those limiting decisions you made long ago—decisions that your conscious mind has forgotten. The unconscious mind ensures that you repeat those old behaviors until you persuade it to adopt a different viewpoint.

How do you talk to your unconscious mind? When you begin to visualize or make up a story, your unconscious mind is involved. When something just pops into your head out of nowhere, that "something" comes from your unconscious mind as well. Having an internal dialog with your rational mind and this other part of you is easy. Try this out. Ask your unconscious mind some questions and just take whatever answer or information jumps into your head first. If you "think" of an answer, that response is coming from your conscious mind! Try asking your unconscious mind these questions and note the answers:

1. How old is this problem I have identified?

2. Is there a purpose for this problem?

3. What is the *one* thing that I don't have or have not yet experienced that if I had that thing or experience would allow the problem to go away?

4. Is my unconscious mind willing to let go of this problem? (Note: It doesn't need to know *how* this will be accomplished, it just needs to be *willing* to release it).

This last question is the most important one, because if your unconscious mind says no to this, you can't really proceed. You can't bludgeon your unconscious mind into submission on this one. If you do happen to get a no response, then adroitly persuade your unconscious mind by reminding it that the *number one* job it has is your survival. You need good eyesight to stay safe in the world! If there is an emotion involved, remind the unconscious mind that anger only raises cholesterol and does bad things to blood pressure. Sadness and depression suppress the immune system. You can be so frozen with fear that you can't act. Usually this is plenty of rationale for the unconscious to be persuaded to let the problem go.

Once you get the go-ahead from your unconscious mind that it is willing to cooperate, you are ready for the Time Dimension Therapy (TDT). Ask your unconscious mind, "When was the *very first time* I experienced this problem?" That could be the first time you ever felt a certain emotion, the first time you decided to limit your eyesight (not see up close or far away, for example), or when you formed a belief or pattern about not seeing clearly. Now, consciously, you don't remember back to early childhood, in the womb, past lives or genealogical events. So, you need to let your unconscious mind just take you on a journey, back as far as it can go until it accesses that first event. You may end up at the first day of school or at your birth. You may go even farther back, past where you can consciously remember, to a past life or the experience of an ancestor. Just let your unconscious mind show you. Make it up! After all, it is your mind that is making it up anyway. Find out if that first event was before you were born, during your birth or after. If it was after your birth, get an age. If it was before, ask if it was in the womb, in a past life or passed down to you from your ancestors. Then pin it down further. What month in the womb? How many generations back in your genealogy? How many past lives back?

Once you have that first event, imagine that you can float up above your life, so you can get a sense of your life being down below you, like a river or a lifeline (a timeline of your life). Whether you see it, sense it, tell yourself about it or get a hazy knowing, any way you do it is just fine. Take yourself back in time along that river of your life to the first event. As you look down on it, notice the following four things:

- Is it night or day? (Remember, *make it up!*)

- Are you alone or with someone?

- What do you have on your feet?

- How are you feeling, and what is happening?

The next step is to look at that first event to see what *"you now"* can see that *"you then"* couldn't. You are bringing all of the resources you have from your life experiences back to that event which occurred so long ago. In a sense, you are mentoring yourself—the "you" of an earlier time in order to see things differently. The idea here is to get the perspective that will allow the "earlier you" to let go of the old emotions surrounding that first event and to remake any decisions that seemed good at the time, but that may have become limiting out in the future. Reframe the situation. Keep the new awareness, the reframed event, and let go of the negative emotions along with any limiting decisions. As a mentor to that "earlier you," you can have higher perspectives and wiser alternatives that the you *then* was too limited, too young or too stuck to have. Use your conscious mind to mentor and teach your unconscious mind to make a new decision or to see things in a new light.

There are two places where you can gain new perspectives and reframe situations. One of these is right at that first event where you can see and feel things about the situation that you could not see at the time the event actually happened. The other place is *before* that first event occurred—before the emotional event and resulting limiting pattern were ever experienced. If you go before that first event in your imagination and you find that the emotion or limiting decision is not there, then you know you have been successful. Getting to a time and place *before the limitation* occurred is the key.

It will literally feel different because there are no limiting beliefs or patterns. If you can still feel the negative emotion and you continue to have the limiting pattern, you probably need to go further back. Just tell your unconscious mind to go well back before you ever felt this emotion and had this limitation.

A very good place to gain new perspectives before coming forward in time is to go *well before* that first event. Once you are experientially before the emotions and limitations of that first event, you are free to see the event with new eyes. You will then be able to come forward along your lifeline through that event into the present time with new wisdom that will enable you to make a more empowering decision about seeing clearly. Instead of deciding to limit your eyesight, you might choose to use your "insight" to help protect you. Or you might decide that others around you who love you will help you to see things. You may decide that you can actually trust your eyes. Whatever it takes for you to shift your focus from a perspective of lack to one of empowerment will be personal to you. Only you can find this out. If nothing comes to you spontaneously, make something up. The result will be the same.

The last step is to clear those old emotions and decisions along your lifeline from the beginning all the way up to the present. For some, once you get a new perspective, the shift just happens automatically. For others, it is like highlighting your lifeline to edit in the positive changes. You can see two rubber bands, one representing the old way and the other representing the new way. Let go of the old-way rubber band while taking hold of the new-way rubber band. Allow the new rubber band to pull you forward along your lifeline, a bit like water skiing. Let it install the new updates in your life as if it is installing a brand new program on your computer. Or you might choose to imagine a snowplow that is powerfully clearing your lifeline of all of its old limitations. You may want to stop at a few significant events on the way back to the present to gain a heightened awareness and additional insights before moving on.

Once back in the present, you will want to see what has changed or shifted. Notice if those old emotions and decisions are still there or if they are *gone now*. Has your eyesight changed at all? What about your emotions? Your view of life? Your relationship to seeing? Throughout this process you are rewriting the stories, the internal representations for who you are. By clearing out those old patterns, you are allowing yourself to respond to your environment afresh rather than looking through the grid of old emotions. You are giving yourself the tools to "be in the now." You are erasing old stimulus-response patterns that kept you recreating the same frumpy shirt pattern no matter which new material you used. Even if the change is something small, like "The world seems a little brighter," it means you were successful.

Change can be a gradual process, coming on as you increase your rapport and trust with your unconscious mind and your eye-brain connection. Workshop participants frequently experience some shift in their eyesight with this process. Some people experience a sense of well-being and empowerment, even though they may not see a change in their eyesight immediately. Others feel a sense of integration, as if their right and left brain hemispheres want to work together, with both of their eyes seeing equally. Some report that they feel a change was made even if they cannot quite put their finger on what it was.

This process is a simplified version of a Time Dimension Therapy technique. It is intended for you to have an experience of being able to shift your state and/or physiology by shifting your Internal Representations. You may be able to make lasting, dramatic changes. You may be able to make baby steps, small incremental improvements. The important point is that you are beginning to make friends with your unconscious mind. You are also beginning to experience how your brain works and how you can change it to transform your life experience. This "getting to know yourself" is an ongoing process; take whatever happens as positive, as you gently develop skill in doing this.

DAILY EYE YOGA

CHAPTER 24

THE DAILY ROUTINE

Eye Yoga is primarily designed to bring your visual habits to consciousness. Your enhanced awareness can help you practice good habits, repeating them until they become the new, more conscious behavior. In doing this, you build new neurological patterns in your mind. Therefore, the time you spend doing the exercises is not as important as the vision habits you are able to improve, integrating them into your normal day.

This part extrapolates the essential descriptions from section 1, where you worked with a partner, to make them readily available for you to do the exercises by yourself on a daily basis. If you need to review a procedure, check back to section 1. Since Eye Yoga needs to be done frequently as it becomes a lifelong program, just as keeping physically fit by regular gym and yoga workouts, we are trying to make it as easy as possible for you. As our dad would say, take away any excuses for not doing it!

When you go to the gym or do yoga, you need to do it on more than one occasion. If you do it only once, you know your results may only be a little soreness. But when you do it over and over, you can deepen the stretches and build strength. Your eyes are like that. When you do stretches for your eyes, it makes them more mobile and flexible, and you can actually begin to see better.

Following are relaxation exercises that can be done during the day to take mini-breaks from extended close work or tension build-up. They can also be done before doing your Eye Yoga routine. Doing these frequently teaches your eyes the good habits of relaxation, breathing, blinking and not staring.

- **Breathe:** Inhale deeply and then exhale twice as long, making a sighing sound. Relax your body as you breathe.

- **Blink:** Blinking regularly moisturizes and massages your eyes, to keep them healthy and reduce staring.

- **Twist and Swing:** Rhythmically twisting your upper torso from side to side as you let your arms and eyes swing along relaxes and stretches the body.

- **Head and Neck Rotations:** Gently roll your head in a circle, clockwise and then reversed, breathing deeply and slowly.

- **Cross-Crawl:** Step in place, raising each knee and touching it with the palm of the other hand to get the right and left brain in sync.

Now you are ready for Eye Yoga! Again we repeat these words of caution: it is very important not to overdo the exercises. Be aware of when your eyes have had enough. Rome wasn't built in a day, as they say. You'd rather have your eyes be as eager as a dog to be taken for a walk than dreading an arduous workout.

CLOCK CIRCLES

Imagine a large clock in front of you. As you breathe fully and easily, look up to 12:00. Sweep your eyes just like a second hand, slowly and smoothly, around the perimeter of the clock, while keeping your head still. Using your finger gives your eyes something to follow. Keep your finger a comfortable distance from your face. Then reverse the direction, doing it several times, clockwise and counterclockwise, adjusting the circle size and the speed to provide a comfortable workout. At first your clock will probably be smaller. As you practice this, you can expand the size of your clock.

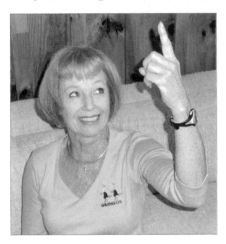

Notice any place where your eyes seem to skip, jump, pause or in any way go out of the smooth rhythm, remembering the areas your partner helped you feel. You may go back to some areas that didn't feel smooth or that your partner had pointed out in order to practice them by doing small arcs back and forth.

Variations

- Move your finger from upper right to lower left on a diagonal, then lower right to upper left. Next, go from side to side, letting your eyes track your finger movements.

- Move your eyes in a Z-formation, a triangle, and a square, using your finger for a guide.

- Make Figure 8s horizontally, vertically and near-to-far. The Figure 8 is easy to do during the day, "on the fly" as it were, whenever you have a minute to stretch your eyes. In the beginning, you may use your finger to trace the Figure 8, giving your eyes a target. Once you can do this, advance to making the figures without a finger to follow.

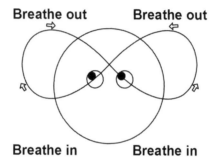

End this warm-up with palming your eyes to relax and rest them.

FINGER PUSH-UPS

Start with a few deep breaths, relaxing and imagining the oxygen going to your eyes. Hold your index finger at arm's length from the tip of your nose, focusing on it as you bring the finger closer and closer to the end of your nose. Now "trombone-slide" your finger back out, concentrating on keeping it in focus. Keep the eyes moving smoothly without jumps or glitches. Feel each one doing its part. Remember any feedback your partner gave you, such as one eye not seeing as actively as the other. Don't let one eye skate by without working! If one eye feels weaker or less engaged, first cover the stronger eye and do the push-ups with the weaker eye to strengthen it. Then do the push-ups again with both eyes.

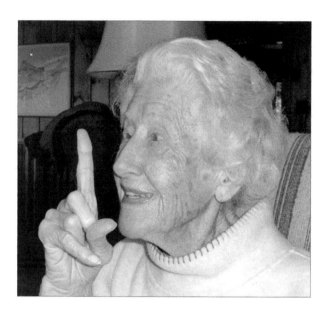

Repeat this slow in-out motion 5–8 times, or fewer, if you feel the stretch and have the sensation that your eyes have gotten a nice workout. Then cup your palms over your closed eyes to relax them.

Journaling

You might want to keep a journal of any changes in your ability to process, such as any right- and left-brain functioning differences, as we discussed earlier. Notice if analytical, numerical and logical tasks become easier. Notice if what were emotional challenges become easier, if a sports activity improves, if your intuition increases or if underlying emotions of fear, anxiety, depression or anger recede in intensity.

"Most men equate journaling to diaries…and let's face it gents, real men don't do diaries. That said, anyone who is striving to make positive change in their life will benefit from a journal. As an endurance athlete, I am a voracious reader of various training techniques and the latest and greatest training aids. There is almost too much information out there. We are all different and there is not a one size fits all answer for anything.

"I keep a training journal to help me with the inevitable trial and error that I face as I work to be the best athlete I can be. The journal helps me to plan and reflect. It's nothing fancy or complex, but contains the necessary information about the workouts and the things going on with and around me. As I am working through a training season or putting a training plan together, I can look back to see what worked in the past and what didn't. If I get injured or off track, I can look back to when I was in a similar position…What caused it… How long did it take to work through it…What did I do to speed or slow the process? I revisit my best and worst results and see what was going on with my life. I assess how it all fit together and use it to tweak my future plan accordingly… you get the idea. It takes just 10 minutes a day and can make a huge difference in your future progress.

"Since I have been working with Jane, I include my visualization work in my journal. It is an integral part of what I do. I can review what specific techntiques I used for any given situation and how I responded. Whether you are looking to improve athletic performance through visualization, looking to heal a physical ailment or seeking to improve your vision, a journal will speed the process and leave you with a wonderful tool for reflection."

—Bond Jones, Austin, Texas

V-IN AND V-OUT

This next exercise is a significant part of your Eye Yoga workout where your eyes are encouraged to work together to create a kind of "double vision." It encourages depth perception.

V-In

Hold your index and middle fingers out in front of you spread into a V shape. Hold the V shape at a comfortable distance from your nose in front of you. Slightly cross your eyes so your eyes are focusing on a spot in front of the finger V until you see three fingers. Put your attention on the center one. Clearly see the tip where the two fingers come together.

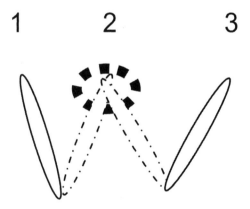

V-Out

Hold your index finger and middle finger out in front of you in a V shape, fingers spread. Look through and past your fingers to the distance until you see three fingers. You may have to adjust how far in the distance you look to make this happen. Experiment with holding your fingers closer or farther away. Once you see the three fingers, put your attention on the center finger. Focus on it. When you have finished, relax by palming for a few minutes.

Jump Vs

Once you can do the V-In and V-Out exercises, you are ready for the expert level. You will move your eyes from convergence to divergence as you go from V-In to V-Out. Eventually, you will be able to jump smoothly and quickly back and forth.

Other Variations

Try the following movements with your fingers as you keep your focus on that "middle finger" of the Vs, with both V-In and V-Out:

In and out like a trombone
Up and down
Right and left
In diagonals
In circles
In Figure 8s

After practicing, relax by palming. Release any tension you feel anywhere in your body.

SEE CIRCLES

This is another way to practice eye convergence and to make both eyes work together.

See In—Convergent SEE Circles

Hold the circles about one to two feet away from your face. Now cross your eyes slightly and look at the space in front of them.

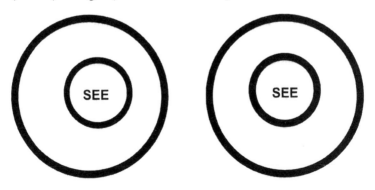

The object is to get your eyes to see three sets of circles. The third set should have the SEEs lined up on top of each other so they look like one. Focus on the middle SEE. If the middle SEEs are not aligned, make sure your head is straight, not tilted to one side.

Practice getting the three circle sets a number of times. When you have finished, relax by palming for a few minutes.

See Out—Divergent SEE Circles

Once you can hold the basic convergence circles, move to diverging your eyes. Look at the two sets of circles again. This time look *beyond* them until you again see three sets. Focus on the SEE in the middle set as before until you can SEE it clearly. If you have trouble making three circles this way, bring the circles up close to your nose and look through them into the distance. Push them away from your face slowly, continually looking far, until three circles are there. Once the middle circles are clear, find the closer circle. This time the inner circle should look closer and the outer circle farther away. That is how you can tell whether your eyes have converged or diverged.

Circle Jumps—Alternating Convergence and Divergence

To try the next level, you will first converge your eyes, making the inner circle farther away. Then you will diverge your eyes to make the inner circle closer. You will be going from SEE In to SEE Out. Eventually you will be able to jump back and forth smoothly and quickly. You can do the same variations with the Circles as with the Vs. By printing the circles from appendix A on clear plastic, you can carry them with you to practice during the day.

KNOTS ON A STRING

The string exercise builds on what you have practiced in V-In, V-Out and in SEE Circles. Use the knotted string you and your partner had. Attach one end of the knotted string to a chair, window, doorknob or dresser so it is just below eye level with nothing to distract your view of the string.

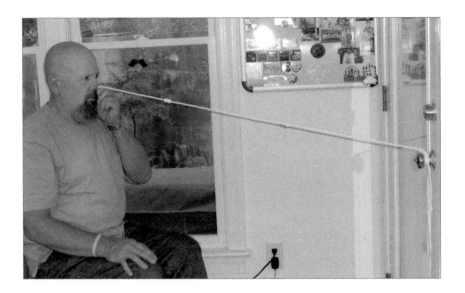

Hold the other end up to or just under your nose. Keep good posture, not leaning over or jutting the head forward to meet the string. Focusing on one knot at a time, see two strings forming an X with one knot in the middle. Practice with knots at different distances.

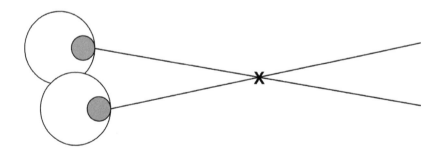

If you have difficulty getting an X through the knot, refer back to the string exercise with a partner in section 1, chapter 8 for more troubleshooting suggestions.

PATCHING

When patching, it is important to be in a safe environment that fosters exploration and experimentation (not while driving). Buy an eye patch, usually found in drug stores, that fits so the covered eye will still be open, but in the dark. Or you can take two pairs of glasses and tape over the right in one and the left in the other.

Patch one eye for up to 20 minutes at a time. Start with 5–10 minutes and work up. Then patch the other eye. You may want to keep a journal or make some notes about what you experience with each eye separately. Sometimes the world will look brighter or darker with one eye. Make note of any emotions that come up. Walk around and take in the environment. Experiment with different activities such as: reading, personal conversations, doing detailed figures or banking, sitting quietly, listening to music, preparing dinner, and walking outside in nature, doing creative arts, crafts or writing. Notice any body sensations, emotions, or mind chatter/thoughts that are there. Many find their right eye to be more left-brained, yang, logical and detailed, and the left eye to be more right-brained, yin, emotional, intuitive and global. Experiment with your own eyes to see what is true for you.

PALMING

Now that you are winding down your Eye Yoga workout, it is time to move to the more relaxing exercises. Even though you did short palming between the exercises, do a longer one at the end to relax your eyes, optic nerves and whole nervous system. Just as you would with your body muscles, it is important to teach your eye muscles to relax.

SUNNING

Sunning is a way to bathe your whole eyeball in light, by closing your eyes and letting the light come through your eyelids. Light is a nutrient. It is necessary for good eye health. We habitually use our eyes in limited patterns that don't get light to all areas of the eyeball. Like lying in the sun at the beach, Sunning your eyes relaxes them and loosens accumulated eye tensions.

Sunning is done with the eyes closed.

Stand in front of a light source, preferably the sun. Gently close your eyes and breathe fully and easily in a regular rhythm. Move your head in an arc, starting with your nose pointing at one shoulder. Raise it up high, turning and pointing it down to the other shoulder. Do this slowly and gently without excessive stretching or strain. Adjust the arc so it is comfortable for you.

Flicker Variation

While you are Sunning, move the outstretched fingers of each hand back and forth over each other to create a flicker on your closed eyelids, like a strobe light. This stimulates the pupils as well as the brain.

PALMING/SUNNING COMBO

This exercise stimulates the pupils to open and close quickly and completely in response to changes in light intensity. Face the sun (or other light source) and begin Sunning in a smooth, relaxed way *with your eyes closed.* Do this for a few minutes. Next, cover your eyes and palm them. Remember to maintain your full, easy breathing. Do this for the same amount of time, or longer, as you did the Sunning. Sometimes it's nice to turn away from the sun to get some darkness. Turn back to the sun for more sun bathing, then away and palm for the soothing darkness. Repeat for as long as you wish and enjoy the relaxed, alert feeling this brings to your eyes and whole nervous system.

VISUALIZATION COOL-DOWN

We've extensively explained the ways in which our thoughts affect our vision, and how the way we see relates to how we think. This cool-down period is a time to explore your inner vision as well as how you see yourself. The better you get to know yourself and befriend your innermost thoughts, the healthier you will become. For this part, after you have done your Eye Yoga exercises, put on some soothing music, a visualization tape or enjoy the silence as you move inward. Some benefits of this process are as follows:

- Mood enhancer, see things in a new light.

- Activate creativity, envisioning new possibilities.

- Suggestibility to your eyes for better vision, your eye-brain-body coordination, new flexibility, etc. Similar to self-hypnosis, you open a communication door to your unconscious mind and to your autonomic nervous system into which you can drop many wonderful suggestions, and change old habits.

- Parasympathetic Nervous System Activation: involves digestion, nourishing, repair, decreasing hormonal output, elimination of waste and toxins and elimination of emotional "plaque." It keeps the body in good functioning order and balances out the tensions of the Sympathetic Nervous System (fight-or-flight and focus). Creates the deep relaxation that comes with the slower brain waves of the alpha state, easing and eliminating tensions and stress.

Some suggestions for using this time are as follows:

- Envision new possibilities in your life, family, society, and the world.

- Enjoy an expanded flow of creativity. Allow new connections, ideas and possibilities to bubble up within you, whether they are innovations or solutions to some problem you are working on.

- Ask your heart how you are really feeling about particular situations that are going on in your life. Ask each eye how it views the situation, then shift into harmony and balance.

- Go to your favorite place and explore it with perfect vision using all of the good habits you have learned. Maybe you love walking on the beach or through a deep, green forest. Let your imagination guide you.

- Breathe calmly and deeply while visualizing happy, healthy eyes.

- Practice various combinations of breathing, palming, listening to soothing music, repeating encouraging words or affirmations that will support your vision, and/or playfully imagining many situations and environments where your vision is perfect.

- In your imagination, explore the joy of having total freedom from glasses or contacts.

- Engage in fun, encouraging conversations with each eye in turn, and then both together, as a happy team working together harmoniously.

- Breathe the colors of the rainbow into your eyes and through your whole body one color at a time and feel the responses to this nourishment and healing.

- Alternate deep breaths and butterfly-like, fluttering blinks with soft eyes.

- Practice performance. Olympic athletes often visualize their performance before competition. Just as someone who wants to lose weight visualizes his or her slim body, you can use this time to visualize your eyes seeing as perfectly as you desire.

- Visualize your eyes performing perfectly for you in a favorite sport, such as tennis or golf, and watch your game improve!

- Use your "imaginal body" to perform various exercises and feats.

RECHECK YOUR VISION

Periodically re-check your vision to see if there has been an improvement. If you see an improvement, congratulations! Watch your long-term trend. Remember, if you see little short-term improvement, don't be concerned. Recall the gym exercises and Pete Cisco's theory that improvement happens *after* the exertion during the recovery period.

CHAPTER 25

WORKOUT PROGRAM

The important thing in doing your Eye Yoga is to do it on a regular basis. While it takes very little time to do and requires almost no equipment (most can be done with your fingers!), it needs to be done daily. Like going to the gym or doing yoga, you need to keep doing it in order to gradually stretch, relax and strengthen the muscles in the eyes and retrain your eye-brain connection. Once your eyes get to a certain level of improvement, you may not have to do the exercises as often. The eyes seem to be trainable in that sense. You may need to go back and do the exercise program on a more regular basis if you feel your eyes slipping back into old patterns of limitation, but once they strengthen, it is possible for them to maintain good vision. At this stage you will have moved from eye exercises into being a partner with a new, healthy, habitual way to use your eyes to see, unifying body and mind, eyesight with internal vision.

Step One is to decide if you will do all of the Eye Yoga exercises or choose specific exercises to do. Below is a checklist you can use, with the date you start each regime. Put the date and an X by whichever exercise regime you choose to do. If you change the regime by adding or dropping any of the exercises, you may want to record that by putting the new date and the appropriate Xs.

EXERCISE REGIME

All Yoga Exercises					
Specific Exercises:					
Circles					
Figure 8s					
Pencil Push-Ups					
V-In, V-Out					
Knots on String					
Palming					
Sunning					
Patching					
Breathing					
Blinking					
Twist & Swing					
Head/Neck Circles					
Cross Crawl					

Step Two is to decide when you will do the exercises. It is suggested that you do the entire regime once a day. Pick a time to do it as part of your daily routine, so it becomes a habit. If you decide, instead, to do some of the exercises only when you have time, "on-the-go," as it were, do them two to six times a day. Choose a time when you can do them as an overlap to something else you do on a regular basis, like brushing your teeth, in the shower, at breakfast or any time you have a few minutes of waiting time. Waiting time can be waiting for an appointment, while you are stuck in traffic (not driving!), waiting for your kids, in line at the supermarket, or any other place where you might otherwise feel you were impatient or wasting time. Some people need help remembering when it is time to do the exercises. Until you get into a routine, you may find it helpful to put reminder notes in strategic places. You could tape a note to your toothpaste or toothbrush, put one in the shower, on your mirror, in your planner, on your to-do list or on the dashboard of your car.

You can choose to do some exercises when you first wake up, before even getting out of bed. The natural light present in the early afternoon makes lunchtime a good time to do Sunning and palming. Patching might be done while engaged in some activity that only requires the use of one eye (vacuuming, cooking, watching TV, putting the kids to bed, making phone calls, preparing a meal or doing chores). Keeping a daily record of your workouts will enable you to track your progress, as well as provide much satisfaction.

Date	Time/ Place	No. Times Daily	Date	Time/ Place	No. Times Daily

HOW LONG SHOULD EACH WORKOUT BE

This depends on how quickly your eyes get tired, how long it takes to give your eyes a good workout, and your unique condition. You should do each exercise only long enough to get a good stretch. Do not overdo it! Maybe 30 seconds of each will be enough to tire you at first. The point is to keep doing the exercises until you can gradually build up to a longer time. ***Overdoing the exercises will not make you see better faster. The regular practice of Eye Yoga over time produces the best results.*** Improvement also depends on how much you have used or rested your eyes, the quality of your nutrition, the amount of sleep you usually get, and so forth. Remember, your vision continuously fluctuates. Some days you may want a lighter workout than on other days because your eyes may be tired. In any case, a little stretching can be good for them. Palming and Sunning can be done to relax them.

EYE YOGA WORKOUT TRACKING

For the full Eye Yoga workout, we suggest specific lengths of time as you first begin practicing each exercise. The entire regimen takes 30–45 minutes. You may want to vary this after a few weeks. For example, you may want to patch for longer periods (20–60 minutes) as you engage in other activities which would be safe for you to do using only one eye. Make the exercises fit your vision goals as well as your routine and incorporate them into your other activities where convenient. In other words, we have given you an Eye Yoga workout routine which contains all of the exercises, but you may well choose to integrate them into your unique schedule and lifestyle.

The Warm-ups and visualizing cool-downs can be done for as long as you like.

Eye Yoga times are guidelines. ***Do not overdo and strain.*** Listen to your eyes and relax between exercises.

ON-THE-GO EYE YOGA

Fit these in wherever you can:

Breathe

Blink

Twist and Swing

Head and Neck Rotations

Clock Circles

Figure 8s,

Finger Push-Ups

V-In, V-Out

Palming

Sunning

Palm/Sun Combo

Visualizing

ADDITIONAL KEY POINTS
TO ACHIEVING GOOD VISION

In addition to the regular Eye Yoga exercises, here are some other key points to remember. We have discussed these earlier in the book, but let us review them here as they are very important.

1. Remember to tell your eyes to "SEE." Tell your brain to focus, relax and *see*. Keep extending the time that they focus and you notice things becoming clearer for an instant. Eventually you will be able to see clearly for longer periods of time.

2. Whenever possible, be aware of your peripheral vision. This can be particularly helpful in driving, playing sports or walking, whether in a crowded area or out in nature. It is also useful to increase the clarity of near vision.

3. Make sure you are getting enough chromium. Nutritionally speaking, monitor and lower your intake of sugars and simple carbohydrates which can deplete chromium. Be sure you are getting enough protein in your diet. Avoid refined foods, heavily-fried foods and overeating. Vitamins needed are A, Bs, C, D and E.

4. Train your eyes and body to be more aware of spatial relation-ships, especially the space between objects both near and far. Notice where you are and be conscious of your relationship to the space around you.

5. If you have glasses or contacts, only use them when necessary, and wean yourself away from using them constantly, as you can do this safely. You can see more than you think, even if your vision is blurry. Seeing without lenses helps you see where you are in space better.

6. Whenever you are doing close work, regularly look away. Rest your eyes and stretch your body. Look out the window or into natural light. Doing this every few minutes is beneficial to break and replace that habitual, turned-in posture with a more relaxing turned-out variation. This also provides welcome respite to eyes craving stimulus variety. And of course, be aware peripherally as you focus.

7. Fight pattern deprivation by varying the distances you are seeing. If you spend extended time doing close work, then frequently look away, focus in the distance. Close your eyes, palm, and do sun-strobing (the flickers "wake up your brain"). Twist and stretch, allowing your eyes to float freely instead of focusing, is good. Keep your eyes moving and blinking, avoiding the frozen stillness of staring.

SPECIFIC BENEFITS FOR EACH EXERCISE

Exercise	Circles	Patching	Finger Push-Ups	V-In, V-Out	Knots on a String	Palming	Sunning
Astigmatism	X		X			X	X
Better Brain Functioning	X	X	X	X		X	X
General Eye Health	X	X	X	X	X	X	X
Light Sensitivity						X	X
Nearsighted Myopia	X	X		V-Out	X	X	X
Presbyopia Farsighted	X	X	X	V-In	X	X	X

261

EYESIGHT TRACKING SHEET

Date	Far Chart Distance	Far Line Read	Near Chart Distance	Near Line Read	Notes

Eye Yoga Routine Workout Tracking Sheet

	Minutes	Record	Date							
			Day	1	2	3	4	5	6	7
Warm – ups	**4**									
• Breathe	½	Minutes or √								
• Blink	½	Minutes or √								
• Twist & Swing	1	Minutes or √								
• Head & Neck	1	Minutes or √								
• Cross Crawl	1	Minutes or √								
Eye Yoga	**18**									
• Clock Circles	2	Minutes or √								
• Figure 8s	2	Minutes or √								
• Finger Push Ups	1	Minutes or √								
• Palm	¼	Minutes or √								
• V in, V out	2	√ or J or V								
• Any Warm – up	¼	Minutes or √								
• See In – See Out	2	√ or J or V								
• Palm	¼	Minutes or √								
• Knots on a String	2	√ or Combo								
• Any Warm – up	¼	Minutes or √								
• Patching	2	Minutes or √								
• Palming	2	Minutes or √								
• Sunning	2	Minutes or √								
Or										
• Palm/Sun Combo (20 sec turns)	4	Minutes or √								
Visualizing Cool Down	**8–23**									
• Visualization	8–23	Minutes or √								

CHAPTER 26

CONCLUSION—AUTHORS' NOTE

We hope you have enjoyed this excursion into Eye Yoga and the relationship between your eyes and your brain; between how you see and how you think. Like pulling a nub of yarn sticking out of a sweater and then finding you are unraveling the whole garment, we hope this book has led you to consider new ideas, connections and possibilities. Your eyes are much more than they might seem at first sight. Your mind creates your reality as a visual fabrication from electrical and chemical signals of light on the retina. Inward sight and insight mold what we see and how we see and believe. Our ability to envision greater possibilities, pulls, motivates and aligns our potential, our behavior and our achievements. This book is really about how simple eye exercises can reawaken deep brain capacities.

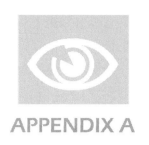

CHARTS

FAR SIGHT CHART

E

B D R

F X O P T S

E N C W A B D

M Q F U R P S G

A O B L S F D T R M

J D T B F Q X Z P S G A R

NEAR SIGHT CHART

Now measure your nearsightedness by reading the lines below. How many lines down can you read?

1. I must be a sight for sore eyes! Good site is all in location.

2. Good sight is in the eye of the beholder. Behold how good my sight is, for I am actually reading this.

3. Good sight is in the eye of the beholder. Behold how good my sight is, for I am actually reading this. I must be a sight for sore eyes! Good site is all in location.

4. Good sight is in the eye of the beholder. Behold how good my sight is, for I am actually reading this. I must be a sight for sore eyes! Good site is all in location.

5. Behold how good my sight is, for I am actually reading this. Good sight is in the eye of the beholder. I must be a sight for sore eyes! Good site is all in location.

6. Good sight is in the eye of the beholder. Behold how good my sight is, for I am actually reading this. I must be a sight for sore eyes! Good site is all in location.

7. Good sight is in the eye of the beholder. I must be a sight for sore eyes! Behold how good my sight is, for I am actually reading this. Good site is all in location.

8. Good sight is in the eye of the beholder. Behold how good my sight is, for I am actually reading this. I must be a sight for sore eyes! Good site is all in location.

9. Good sight is in the eye of the beholder. Behold how good my sight is, for I am actually reading this. I must be a sight for sore eyes! Good site is all in location.

10. Good sight is in the eye of the beholder. Behold how good my sight is, for I am actually reading this. I must be a sight for sore eyes! Good site is all in location.

11. Good sight is in the eye of the beholder. Behold how good my sight is, for I am actually reading this. I must be a sight for sore eyes! Good site is all in location.

12. Good site is all in location. Good sight is in the eye of the beholder. Behold how good my sight is, for I am actually reading this.

EYESIGHT TRACKING SHEET

Date	Far Chart Distance	Far Line Read	Near Chart Distance	Near Line Read	Notes

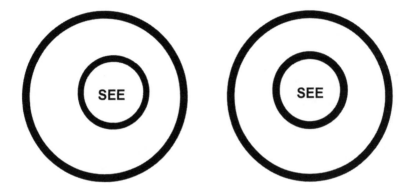

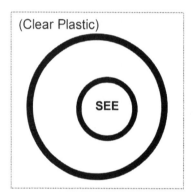

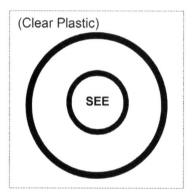

Eye Yoga Routine Workout Tracking Sheet

	Minutes	Record	Date							
			Day	1	2	3	4	5	6	7
Warm–ups	**4**									
• Breathe	½	Minutes or √								
• Blink	½	Minutes or √								
• Twist & Swing	1	Minutes or √								
• Head & Neck	1	Minutes or √								
• Cross Crawl	1	Minutes or √								
Eye Yoga	**18**									
• Clock Circles	2	Minutes or √								
• Figure 8s	2	Minutes or √								
• Finger Push Ups	1	Minutes or √								
• Palm	¼	Minutes or √								
• V in, V out	2	√ or J or V								
• Any Warm–up	¼	Minutes or √								
• See In – See Out	2	√ or J or V								
• Palm	¼	Minutes or √								
• Knots on a String	2	√ or Combo								
• Any Warm–up	¼	Minutes or √								
• Patching	2	Minutes or √								
• Palming	2	Minutes or √								
• Sunning	2	Minutes or √								
Or										
• Palm/Sun Combo (20 sec turns)	4	Minutes or √								
Visualizing Cool Down	**8–23**									
• Visualization	8–23	Minutes or √								

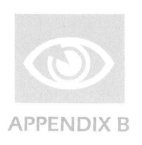

PERSONALITY TESTS

Want to find out more about yourself? Below are two tests you can take. Take the first test to determine whether your predominant way of processing is visual, auditory or kinesthetic, and discover ways in which people can talk to you to really get your attention. The second test, similar to the Myers-Briggs Test, gives your personality profile.

TEST 1

Find your Preferred Representational System—Visual, Auditory, Kinesthetic or Auditory-Digital: We take in and process information through our five senses. Each of us has preferred ways of doing this—visually (primarily through pictures), auditorily (through sounds), kinesthetically (through emotions, sensations and feelings), and through our sense of taste and smell. A sixth way of processing, called auditory-digital, is analytical, usually involving talking to oneself. To find out your preferred way of processing (called your Representational System), take the test below.

Why would you want to know? You can learn more about yourself, what kind of language appeals to you, what kind of people just seem to be more likeable to you. People who have the same

Representational System will seem more familiar to you, as if you are speaking the same language. You may feel as if you've known them before or they may remind you of someone. You may find you have an instant rapport with them. When you want someone to like you, when you want to speak to them in their own language, or when you want to influence someone, it is useful to know that person's preferred processing style.

Take a Test: Here is a very simple test to find your preferred Representational System. For each of the following statements, put a number next to every phrase, using the following system: Put numbers in the blanks beside all of the answers. Every blank needs a number.

Closest to describing you	=	4
Next best description	=	3
Next best	=	2
Least descriptive of you	=	1

1. I make important decisions based on:
   ___ gut level feelings.
   ___ which way sounds the best.
   ___ what looks best to me.
   ___ precise review and study of the issues.

2. During an argument, I am most likely to be influenced by:
   ___ the other person's tone of voice.
   ___ whether or not I can see the other person's argument.
   ___ the logic of the other person's argument.
   ___ whether or not I feel I am in touch with the other person's true feelings.

3. I most easily communicate what is going on with me by:
   ___ the way I dress and look.
   ___ the feelings I share.

___ the words I choose.

___ the tone of my voice.

4. It is easiest for me to:

___ find the ideal volume and tuning on a stereo system.

___ select the most intellectually relevant point concerning an interesting subject.

___ select the most comfortable furniture.

___ select rich, attractive color combinations.

5.

___ I am very attuned to the sounds of my surroundings.

___ I am very adept at making sense of new facts and data.

___ I am very sensitive to the way articles of clothing feel on my body.

___ I have a strong response to colors and to the way a room looks.

Now, copy your answers from the test to the lines below:

1. ___ K	2. ___ A	3. ___ V	4. ___ A	5. ___ A
___ A	___ V	___ K	___ D	___ D
___ V	___ D	___ D	___ K	___ K
___ D	___ K	___ A	___ V	___ V

Add the numbers associated with each letter. (There should be 5 entries for each letter). In other words, looking at column 1 above, copy the number you put beside K in the K column below. Copy the number beside A in the A column below. Then copy the number by V in the V column below, and so on. Transfer the numbers in each of the five columns above to the four columns below.

V	K	A	D
———	———	———	———
———	———	———	———
———	———	———	———
———	———	———	———
———	———	———	———
Totals ———	———	———	———

Totals: Add the numbers in each of the columns to get totals. The highest score is the preferred representational system.

FAVORED REPRESENTATIONAL SYSTEMS— DESCRIPTIONS OF THE CATEGORIES

V: Visual

People who are visual often stand or sit with their heads and/or bodies erect, with their eyes up. They will be breathing from the top of their lungs. They often sit forward in their chair and tend to be organized, neat, well-groomed and orderly. They memorize by seeing pictures, and are less distracted by noise. They often have trouble remembering verbal instructions because their minds tend to wander. A visual person will be interested in how your program *looks*. Appearances are important to them. They are often thin and wiry.

A: Auditory

People who are auditory will move their eyes sideways (remember Richard Nixon?). They breathe from the middle of their chest. They typically talk to themselves, and are easily distracted by noise. (Some even move their lips when they talk to themselves). They can repeat things back to you easily, they learn by listening, and usually like music and talking on the phone. They memorize by steps, proce- dures, and sequences. Auditory people like to be *told* how they are doing, and respond to the tone of voice or set of words. They will be interested in what you have to say about your program.

K: Kinesthetic

People who are kinesthetic will typically be breathing from the bottom of their lungs, so you'll see their stomach go in and out when they breathe. They often move and talk verrry slooowly. They respond to physical rewards and touching. They also stand closer to people than a visual person typically would. They memorize by doing or walking through something. They will be interested in your program if it "feels right," or if it is something they can *grasp* or *get a handle on.*

A$_d$: Auditory Digital

These people will spend a fair amount of time talking to themselves. They will want to know if your program "makes sense." The auditory-digital types can exhibit characteristics of the other major representational systems as well. The qualities of the A$_d$ person are ones that are encouraged by our society, not necessarily ones we are born with. To find your true Rep System, you may want to take out the A$_d$ scores to see whether visual, auditory or kinesthetic gets the highest score.

Adapted from and used with permission, copyright © 1987, 1994 Tad James and Advanced Neuro Dynamics.

REFERENCE BOOKS

The Magic of NLP Demystified—Byron Lewis and Frank Pucelik

Frogs into Princes—Richard Bandler, John Grinder

Therapeutic Metaphors—David Gordon

TEST 2

The second test, based on the Myers-Briggs Test, the Keirsey-Bates book, *Please Understand Me,* and Tad James' work with metaprograms tells you about your behavior and what motivates you. Then there is a section on what all of that means and why it is important. Following that is information about how you can use these simple tests to learn more about yourself. Understanding who you are can lead to a greater empathy and understanding of others. Answer the questions, then look below for a description. Usually people are a mixture, yet these questions force a choice. Choose the one that best fits you.

Extrovert or Introvert? (Your external behavior)

When you want to recharge your batteries, do you prefer to be alone or with others?

Which do you prefer—being outside in the world of activity, things and people or inside with your thoughts, feelings and ideas?

Sensor or Intuitor? (Your internal behavior)

When you study something new, are you more interested in the facts and their utility in the now or are you more interested in the relationships between the ideas and their utility for the future? When you collaborate on a project, are you more interested in getting the job done or the long-range implications of the project?

Feeler or Thinker? (Your internal state)

How would you rather be thought of as:
A fair person? Or a reasonable person?
A caring person? Or a logical person?
A sensitive person? Or a person who's above feelings?

Judger or Perceiver? (Your adaptation operator)

If you were going to do a project or job, would you prefer that it be orderly, sequential and planned ahead of time without changing the plans once made, or would you prefer it be loosely planned to allow more flexibility as you go along? Do you like things decided on beforehand and the plan stuck to, or have a plan with options and "wiggle room" built in?

Extrovert—likes to be with others instead of being alone or with one other person. The extrovert appears to have a need for sociability, often appearing "tuned up" when with people, feeling lonely when not in contact with others. They often enjoy large groups over one-to-one.

Introvert—prefers to be alone to recharge batteries, inside with their thoughts, feelings and ideas, finds being with more than one person at a time to be draining, needing their space, private time. Being "territorial," they can be lonely *in* a crowd.

Sensor—interested in the facts and their utility in the present. Often preferring action to daydreaming, getting things done to mulling over different ideas, often loves details, relates to the world around them, in tune with what and who is in their environment.

Intuitor—interested in the relationships between ideas and their use in the future. May appear dreamy or distracted, not paying attention to the present reality, taking to heart broken promises as breaking of a trust, often seeming to be their own person, displaying passion and a tendency toward deep trust and emotion to those they idealize.

Thinker—reasonable, logical, above feelings. Prefers reasons for being asked to do something, often prefers not to be touched, less swayed by approval or disapproval. Prefers to think things through reasonably and logically rather than emote about them.

Feeler—fair, caring, sensitive. Sensitive to their emotional environment and feelings of others, enjoys listening to happenings of family and friends. Often takes on caring responsibilities for others. Shows emotions and often enjoys touch.

Judger—planned, orderly, sequential, things settled and decided on, chosen and established. Likes things settled, nailed down, so they can be relied upon. Once a decision is made, they prefer not to change it—stick with the plan.

Perceiver—unstructured, flexibility built in so if a new idea comes along, it can be incorporated. Likes options left open. Leave open-endedness for creativity.

We all have filters through which we run everything we take in with our five senses. These filters determine our internal state and our physiology. Those in turn determine our behavior. Our filters include our values, our beliefs, our attitudes, our past memories, and our *metaprograms*. The above test gives you four of your personal metaprograms, through which you filter your life experiences.

Why is this important? Why should you care? Because these metaprograms are the key to understanding your own behavior. If you want to change your behavior, one key is to know your own metaprograms. Here is another reason. Every second, we have two million bits of information coming in at us, bombarding our senses. Now, we can only pay attention to about 126 of those two million bits. Exactly what we pay attention to and what we do with the information is determined in large part by these filters. We can't possibly pay attention to two million bits per second, so we delete some information, we generalize some ("Oh, I know what that is—I've seen it before"), and we distort other data (a dark piece of rope in the path looks like a snake for an instant, or what you *thought* you heard was just what you wanted to hear).

The importance of knowing that we only pay attention to a small portion of information available to our senses and that we delete, distort and generalize that information is that our "reality" isn't reality. It is only "reality" as we have perceived and constructed it. We virtually construct our own internal reality by the things we pay attention to. (Does this sound a little bit like *The Matrix*?) It means we are more in control of our own reality than we may have thought.

OTHER REFERENCES

Please Understand Me—Character and Temperament Types by David Keirsey and Marilyn Bates. (Gives more detail on the Myers-Briggs types from the test above).

Flow by Mihaly Csikszentmihalyi. (Source for the two million bits coming in, 126 taken in).

Time Line Therapy and the Basis of Personality by Tad James and Wyatt Woodsmall. (More on metaprograms, values and Time Line Therapy).

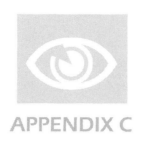

RESOURCES

We have listed some resources that we either know personally or are familiar with to give readers a starting place to find contacts that fit their specific needs. First, we have listed individual contacts, then organizations and websites that can also help.

Natural Vision Improvement Instructors, Behavioral Optometrists, Websites and Product Information Contacts:

Eastern U.S.

Rosemary Gaddum Gordon, D.B.O., M.A.
Holistic Vision Improvement
Cambridge Health Associates
335 Broadway
Cambridge, MA 02139
(617) 354-8360 ext/ 20
and/or
Lightwater
43 Mast Cove Road
Eliot, ME 03903
(207) 439-9821

rosemary@visioneducators.com
http://visioneducators.com
www.cambridgehealthassociates.com/rosemary.html
Specialties: After qualifying as an Orthoptist from Moorfields Eye
Hospital, London, Rosemary added Yoga and the Bates Method
to her practice. Her long interest in issues that sometimes underlie
visual difficulties led her to study Gestalt, Focusing and Eriksonian
hypnotherapy. Combining this with training in Craniosacral and
Self-Regulation Therapy allows for a holistic, in-depth approach to
each individual.

Raymond Gottlieb, O.D., Ph.D.

336 Berkeley Street
Rochester, NY 14607
(585) 461-3716
Florida phone: (727) 367-4851
raygottlieb@frontiernet.net
Specialties: Optometrist specializing in natural vision
improvement, syntonic phototherapy and optometric vision
therapy approaches. Works with myopia, presbyopia, learning
problems, brain injury neurorehabilitation, low vision and
strabismus. Summers are spent at Chautauqua, NY. He frequently
visits the St. Petersburg/Tampa, FL, area and could see vision
students there. Phone sessions are available.

Marc Grossman O.D., LAc

3 Paradise Lane
New Paltz, NY 12561
(845) 255-3728
    and/or
20 Chestnut Street
Rye, NY 10580
(914) 967-1740
www.visionworksusa.com
vision2030@earthlink.net

Martha M. Rigney
363 Meredith St.
Raleigh, NC 27606
(919) 821-0000
eyeyogamartha@gmail.com
Specialties: Natural vision improvement educator, helping people
see connections between their life and their vision to facilitate
improvements in both.

Martin Sussman
Cambridge Institute for Better Vision
65 Wenham Road
Topsfield, MA 01983
(800) 372-3937
(978) 887-3883
marty@bettervision.com
www.bettervision.com
www.withoutglasses.com
www.program-for-better-vision.com

Western U.S.

Neal Apple, M.D.
P.O. Box 5000
Silver City, NM 88062
(575) 523-2020
(575) 521-1553 fax
appleallen1@yahoo.com
Specialties: Board-certified Comprehensive Ophthalmologist and
body-centered psychotherapist trained in Gestalt therapy. Interested in working with clients who want to improve vision and work
on underlying emotional issues.

Samuel A. Berne, O.D.
227 East Palace Avenue, Suite G
Santa Fe, NM 87501

(505) 984-2030
Sberneod@cybermesa.com
www.newattention.net
Specialties: Behavioral Optometry, holistic health, developmental delays in children, cranial sacral therapy, light therapy, nutrition.

Dr. Lee Hartley, Doctorate in Counseling Psychology

401 Alberto Way, Suite1, #3
Los Gatos, CA 95032
(408) 356-0300
Leehartley1@verizon.net
Specialties: A doctorate in Education and a licensed M.F.T. Her therapeutic focus is Post-Traumatic Stress Disorder (PTSD), Anxiety, Depression, and Seasonal Affective Disorder (SAD), utilizing clinical hypnosis, EMDR, Bright White Light Therapy and various forms of biofeedback. She has successfully treated vision issues with some clients.

Dr. Edward Kondrot, M.D. (H), CCH, Dht

2001 Camelback Road, #150
Phoenix, AZ 85015
(800) 430-9328
drkondrot@healingtheeye.com
www.healingtheeye.com
Specialties: Board-certified Ophthalmologist and certified homeopathic doctor, author. He developed an instrument called Microcurrent Stimulator to help improve the vision of people with macular degeneration and glaucoma. It uses a combination of acupuncture and electricity to stimulate healing by increasing retinal circulation, retinal cell metabolism and possibly cell regeneration. 94% of age-related macular degeneration patients experienced increases in visual acuity.

Jacob Liberman, O.D., Ph.D.

Exercise Your Eyes, Inc.
133 Ka Drive

Kula, Hawaii 96790
(Island of Maui)
www.exerciseyoureyes.com
jacob@exerciseyoureyes.com or jacob@jacobliberman.org
Specialties: Author, public speaker, inventor and consultant. Integrates light, vision and consciousness to improve vision and overall performance and to expand awareness. He offers phone consults and ongoing mentoring.

Meir Schneider, Ph.D., LMT
School for Self-Healing
2218 48th Avenue
San Francisco, CA 94116
(415) 665-9574
(415) 665-1318 fax
info@self-healing.org
www.self-healing.org
Specialties: Schneider is the founder of The School for Self Healing, a non-profit school that teaches and provides movement work, massage and vision improvement in San Francisco as well as around the globe for a wide variety of disorders, diseases and injuries. He used the Bates Method to cure himself of congenital blindness and went on to develop the Meir Schneider Method of Self-Healing Through Bodywork and Movement. The technique has been medically documented to help people with Muscular Dystrophy and can help increase mobility, improve the function of body systems, relieve pain, improve vision and increase productivity.

Austria

Dr. Roberto Kaplan
Specialist Consultant in Vision
c/o Fuenkhgasse 11/5
Pressbaum. A-3021
Austria

HYPERLINK "mail:info@beyond2020vision.com"
"http://www.beyond2020vision.com/"
Specialties: In Europe, I offer specialized consultation services for nearsightedness, astigmatism, strabismus, and most importantly, eye disease conditions. With a vast array of medical specialists available for referral, my approaches use psychosomatic methods of dealing with eye problems in children and adults. In addition, I offer courses for professionals to learn my methods. Phone appointments are available.

Australia/New Zealand

Barry Auchettl
Eye Power
Ballarat, Victoria
Australia, 3352
Ph: +61 3 90130232
barry@eyepower.com.au
www.eyepower.com.au
Specialties: Focusing on using muscle testing to see the underlying causes to vision issues. Author of "Eye Power," a 10 minute a day guide to improving your eyesight.

Carina Goodrich
12 Crystal Waters
65 Kilcoy Lane
Conondale, Qld
Australia, 4552
Ph: 61 7 54944888
carina@janetgoodrichmethod.com
janetgoodrichmethod.com
Carina is one of the daughters of Janet Goodrich Ph.D., world renowned author on Natural Vision Improvement and founder of the Janet Goodrich Method. Carina trained with and worked alongside Janet since childhood and offers international live classes via telephone, products for home use to students and class

materials for teachers around the world. Carina also conducts individual and group Vision Retreats, Instructor Training, and Parent/Child Playcamps in The Janet Goodrich Method. Enjoy a FREE 34-minute audio lesson with Carina Goodrich. Download available from www.JanetGoodrichMethod.com. Designed so you can use the activity again and again.

Peter Grunwald
P.O. Box 46325
Herne Bay
Auckland, New Zealand
Ph: +64 (0) 9-360-1730
p.grunwald@clear.net.nz
www.eyebody.com
Specialties: Peter specializes in applying the Alexander Technique principles to improving eyesight and vision. He discovered unique relationships between areas of eyes, the visual pathways and body functions. He leads workshops in the USA, UK, Germany, Switzerland, Australia and New Zealand. He also runs a private practice in Auckland, New Zealand.

Canada

Elizabeth Abraham
Vision Education Centre
339 Bloor Street W., #215
Toronto, Ontario
Canada M5S 1W7
(416) 599-9202
elizabeth@visioneducators.com
www.visioneducators.com

Roberto Kaplan, O.D., M.Ed., FCOVD
Integrated Vision Therapist
Beyond 2020 Vision®
P.O. Box 68

Roberts Creek, British Columbia
Canada V0N 2W0
(206) 905-1393
www.robertokaplan.com
www.kaplaneyecode.eu
www.integratedvisiontherapy.com
info@beyond2020vision.com
http://www.beyond2020vision.com/
Specialties: In supporting people long distance in finding the
root cause of their vision problem as it relates to their life. As a
Board-certified Optometrist in Vision Therapy, I draw on my
scientific training and forty years of experience to guide you in
using specially designed lens prescriptions and training practices
so you can increase the way your eyes function. There is more, so
go to my website.

The Netherlands

Thomas R. Quackenbush
Natural Vision Center
P.O. Box 1241
6501BE Nijmegen
The Netherlands (Holland)
Office: +31 (0) 24 622-2982
Fax: +31 (0) 24 622-2983
From the U.S., dial (011) 3124 622-2982
TomQ@NaturalVisionCenter.com
www.NaturalVisionCenter.com

Worldwide

Jean Houston, Ph.D.
P.O. Box 501
2305-C Ashland St.
Ashland, OR, USA 97520
Office: (541) 488-1200
www.jeanhouston.org
TheOffice@jeanhouston.org

Specialties: As a bestselling author of many books, including *A Mythic Life, The Search for the Beloved, Jump Time* and *A Passion for the Possible,* she is internationally renown as one of the foremost visionary thinkers and doers of our times. As a scholar, philosopher, teacher, and co-director of the Foundation for Mind Research (now the Jean Houston Foundation), she is regarded as one of the principal founders of the Human Potential Movement. She has served in the field of human development in many countries as a consultant to the UN, principally as a consultant to UNICEF, other international agencies and for individual countries. Visit her website, www.jeanhouston.org, for more information on her Mystery Schools, given on the east and west coasts in the U.S., her Social Artistry programs and her visionary quests to "ignite the fires of passionate new ways of becoming our future selves—the future humanity."

ORGANIZATIONS

Association of Vision Educators

Their purpose is to increase public awareness of natural and integrated vision care and encourage education, communication and research in the field. A list of practitioners throughout the world is maintained on their website: www.visioneducators.org.

College of Optometrists in Vision Development

www.covd.org

The College of Optometrists in Vision Development (COVD) is a non-profit, international membership association of eye-care professionals including optometrists, optometry students, and vision therapists. Established in 1971, COVD provides board certification for eye doctors and vision therapists who are prepared to offer state-of-the-art services in:

- Behavioral and developmental vision-care
- Vision therapy
- Visual rehabilitation

These specialized vision-care services develop and enhance visual abilities and correct many vision problems in infants, children, and adults.

Their mission is to serve as an advocate for comprehensive vision care, emphasizing a developmental and behavioral approach. COVD certifies professional competency in vision therapy, serves as an informational and educational resource, and advances research and clinical care in vision development and therapy.

COVD's goal is to facilitate ongoing development in the areas of behavioral and developmental vision care, advocate for wider adoption of vision therapy protocols, and increase recognition of their integral role in enhancing learning, productivity and overall quality of life.

The COVD International Examination and Certification Board process includes a rigorous evaluation of the eye-care professional's knowledge and abilities in providing developmental and behavioral vision care for patients. Optometrists who successfully complete their certification process are Board-certified in Vision Development and Vision Therapy and are designated Fellows of COVD (FCOVD). Vision therapists are certified to work with COVD Fellows as Certified Optometric Vision Therapists (COVT). Vision care provided by all COVD members is based on the principle that vision can be developed and changed. For example, we know that infants are not born with fully developed visual abilities and that good vision is developed through a learned process.

Optometric Extension Program Foundation

1921 E. Carnegie Avenue
Suite 3-L, Santa Ana, CA
USA, 92705-5510
Tel: (949) 250-8070, Fax: (949) 250-8157
www.oep.org

The Optometric Extension Program Foundation, an international organization, is dedicated to the advancement of optometry through the gathering and dissemination of information on vision. Established in 1928 by A. M. Skeffington, the father of behavioral optometry, OEP has 3500 members worldwide. Their mission is to advance human progress through research and education on vision, the visual process, and clinical care. Their goals are to educate optometrists as well as the public about visual health and hygiene, the prevention of visual and ocular problems, understanding of visual development, visual rehabilitation and enhancement of vision and the visual process. They encourage research in these areas and provide education for the discipline of optometry. They also provide access to instruments, equipment, publications and related materials. They promote the post-graduate education of optometrists, with emphasis on behavioral optometry and vision therapy. Their website includes their monthly *Journal of Behavioral Optometry* and reprints of writings and lectures.

College of Syntonic Optometry

Founded in 1933, the College promotes the therapeutic application of light to the visual system. In addition, it supports both public and professional awareness of color light treatment, research in this area, and access to syntonic therapy. It gives an annual conference on light and vision, and workshops are available in the U.S., Great Britain, Europe and Australia. Included are presentations by scientists and clinicians from related fields and basic as well as advanced courses in syntonic phototherapy. To locate a qualified practitioner, visit their active website: www.syntonicphototherapy.com or call: (866) 486-0190.

Their brochure states: "Today, scientific and clinical verification of light's impact on health and healing and a growing public demand for functional and rehabilitative vision therapy continue to vitalize the college and advance its mission."

TIME DIMENSION THERAPY AND TIME LINE THERAPY© THERAPISTS

Jane R. Battenberg, M.A., D.C.H.
3487 San Marino Circle
Costa Mesa, CA, 92626 USA
(714) 556-7858
Email: eyeyogajane@gmail.com
Website: changewithin.com
Specialties: Doctorate in Clinical Hypnotherapy, Neuro-Linguistic Programming Master Trainer. A therapist since 1995, she specializes in changing limiting patterns and negative emotions that manifest in the physical, psychological, metaphysical and spiritual arenas in adults and children. She trains and certifies professionals in Time Dimension Therapy through her company CHANGEWITHIN. Phone sessions are available.

Maggie Connor, D.C.H.
Big Island, HI
(808) 557-5224
Email: maggieconnor@msn.com
Website: maggieconnor.com
Specialties: Neuro-Linguistic Programming Trainer. As an Olympic skier, she works with athletes, high-powered professionals and people who want to make changes to their life patterns and achieve excellence. As a life coach and hypnotherapist, she is available for phone consultations and transformative workshops.

Lorraine K. Flores, Ph.D.
CA, USA
(949) 613-1014
Email: lkf@loriflores.com
Specialties: Doctorate in Clinical Psychology, Neuro-Linguistic Programming Master Trainer, Astrologer. She specializes in changing belief patterns and negative emotions in a person's life,

using astrology and archetypes in conjunction with the therapy for personal change work. Phone sessions are available.

Therese Tappouni, CHT, Time Dimension Therapist
Lance D. Ware, M.A., CHT, Time Dimension Therapist
(888) 77relax (toll free): Tampa, FL offices
Email: Therese@IsisInstitute.org; Lance@IsisInstitute.org
Website: IsisInstitute.org
Specialties: State Bar of CA MCLE Provider in Substance Abuse, Board-certified Clinical and Medical Hypnotherapists, Somatic Intuitive Training™ Practitioners and Trainers, authors, co-founders of Isis Institute. They specialize in emotional intelligence that enhances insight and eyesight via counseling, stress management, and intentional life programs for individuals and organizations since 1990. Phone sessions are available.

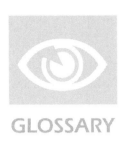

GLOSSARY

Accommodation: The ability of the eye to adjust its focus for near or distance vision, done through the eye lens by relaxing or tightening the ciliary muscle. To see up close, you increase accommodation; and to see far, you relax accommodation.

Aim: Direct the eyes at a target.

Astigmatism: The situation where a point of focus cannot be made on the retina. (The root is the Greek word meaning "without a point.") The refraction of light is uneven in different meridians, so lines in one direction may be blurred while in other directions may not be. Possibly caused by emotional stresses, poor posture and physical conditions.

Bates Method: A system developed by ophthalmologist William Bates, M.D., based on his theory that stress, particularly mental stress, and lack of attention, cause most eye problems. He had many ways to improve vision, including relaxation, eye exercises and visualizations, emphasizing the relationship between body and mind, freeing people from dependence on glasses and professionals.

Behavioral Optometry: A specialized branch of optometry where the doctors are trained in the entire developmental process of vision, so their approach is to build on these visual skills in their work with patients. They don't just provide glasses; they take in all the visual skills in retraining a person how to see. This may extend to influences on eyesight such as environment, posture, nutrition, and general health. Treatment often involves vision therapy.

Binocular Vision: When both eyes work and see together, the result is clear images and depth perception.

Ciliary Muscles: The muscles encircling the lens, contracting and relaxing to change its shape. This allows us to focus near (contract) or far (relax).

Converge, convergence: When the two eyes move toward each other in order to focus on a near object. The eyes point inward (nasally, medially) in order to see up close.

Cornea: The transparent front surface of the eye, covering the iris and the pupil, and whose curvature is responsible for three-fourths of the refraction in the eye.

Cones: The photoreceptive cells in the retina responsible for central vision, color vision and detail that require illumination (light) to see.

Corpus Callosum: The thick band of commissural fibers that connects the right and left cerebral hemispheres of our brain.

Diverge, divergence: When the two eyes move away from each other in order to focus at a distance. They appear to point straight ahead as they move temporally, away from the nose.

Extraocular Muscles: The six muscles, attached to the outside of the eyeball, that turn the eye in, out, up, down and around.

Eye Accessing Patterns: When a person accesses different representational systems in their brain, the eyes move in certain directions. Moving the eyes in these specified directions aids in processing and retrieving visual, auditory or kinesthetic information.

Farsighted (hyperopia): You can see clearly at a distance but not up close. The focus point is behind the retina when accommodation is fully relaxed.

Focus: The point where light rays passing through the cornea and lens meet, on the foveal part of the retina, making an object appear clear.

Fovea: A small depression near the center of the retina where the image is focused by the lens and where most of the cones are concentrated.

Fusion: The brain's ability to blend together the messages coming from each eye.

Internal Representations: The way we represent pictures, sounds, feelings, taste and smell (our five senses) inside our brains. Our sensory experiences and memories are stored in our brains' visual, auditory, kinesthetic, gustatory and olfactory receptors.

Iris: The colored part of the eye surrounding the black pupil opening, made up of connective tissue, muscles and pigmentation. The iris regulates the size of the pupil's opening.

Left brain: The left hemisphere of the brain, associated with logic, analysis, language and reason.

Lens: The transparent, flexible part of the eye, behind the pupil, that changes shape to focus light. Responsible for one-fourth of the light's refraction onto the retina. Also used to describe eye glasses, contacts and implanted lenses (as after cataract surgery).

Macula: An oval, yellowish pit in the center of the retina. Its center is the fovea, where vision is the keenest.

Myopic: Nearsighted.

Nearsighted (myopia): Able to see well up close, but seeing at a distance is blurry. The focus point is in front of the retina when accommodation is increased. A refractive area where the eyeball is too long, the cornea too curved, or the lens unable to relax.

Neuro-Linguistic Programming (NLP): NLP is a series of techniques and methodologies formulated in the 1970s by John Grinder and Richard Bandler to show how our brain stores, processes and retrieves information and how that affects our state of mind (feelings, emotions) and our behavior.

NLP outlines the ways in which the brain creates and stores our subjective experiences. NLP seeks to describe our thinking process and how it determines our feelings and behavior. It works with the *structure*, not the *content*, of these subjective experiences. It analyzes the ways in which we witness our own thinking, and examines how our observations produce various behaviors and states. In this sense, we are not looking at reality, but at the way in which we construct or *experience* reality! (The map is not the territory). NLP shows us *how* our perceptions of reality are created internally. As a form of transpersonal psychology, it provides tools and techniques for removing undesirable patterns, behaviors and states of mind.

Neurotransmitters: Chemical substances in the body that transmit nerve impulses across a synapse between neurons. They include hormones, peptides and opiates.

Ophthalmologist: A medical doctor (M.D). specializing in eye health and disease and able to perform surgeries. This is the doctor you would see if you have a serious eye injury or an eye disease requiring surgery. Ophthalmologists can also prescribe glasses or contacts.

Optician: A person who makes, fits and adjusts glasses, and in some states also fits contact lenses, for lens prescriptions written by optometrists and ophthalmologists.

Optometrists: State-licensed eye-care professionals, able to examine and diagnose eyes, treat some eye diseases and vision disorders, prescribe glasses, contacts, vision therapy, medication and low-vision rehabilitation, and perform some minor surgeries.

Pinhole Glasses: These are glasses made of black opaque plastic lenses that have a series of pinholes in them through which the person can see. First invented by Leonardo da Vinci, they allow the wearer to experience clearer vision without lenses. They are a transition tool to wear for TV, movies or reading instead of regular glasses to reduce the recovery time when one is transitioning to less lens wear.

Presbyopia: The gradual hardening of the eye lens, causing it to become more inflexible and unable to accommodate (change focus) or to see up close. Often associated with getting older.

Retina: The part of the eye located at the back inside of the eyeball that translates the light image into electrical impulses which are then sent to the brain through the optic nerve.

Right brain: The right side of the brain associated with orientation in space, artistry, face recognition, sensuality, holistic, intuitive and big-picture thinking.

Suppression: The brain shuts off part or all of the information (image, movement, color) from one eye. Suppression occurs periodically during the day in the average person, depending on their needs, fatigue and stress levels and what is going on situationally. Since it takes effort and energy and over time could drive a person to some deeper form of adaptation, reducing suppression will bring a more efficient, binocular way of seeing.

Time Dimension Therapy: A therapy based on Neuro-Linguistic Programming models that uses visualization (a person's internal representations of visual, auditory, kinesthetic, gustatory and olfactory) to reprogram the unconscious mind to change behavior, negative emotions, limiting beliefs and repeating patterns in a person's life that they want to change.

Vision Therapy: A therapy program for the eyes used primarily by behavioral optometrists that makes the person aware of what the eyes are doing and teaches them to improve their visual skills (see Behavioral Optometry). Since vision is learned and developed sequentially, Vision Therapy fills in the missing skills. The targeted results are not only improved vision but improvement in other areas, a few of which are learning facility, interactive and socialization skills, conceptualization, visualization, and creativity.

Visual Acuity: The sharpness of one's vision or sight; how close to 20/20 your vision is. The ability to discern small details.

BIBLIOGRAPHY AND
SUGGESTED READING

Agarwal, Dr. R. S. *Yoga of Perfect Sight.* Pondicherry, India: Sri Auribundo Ashram, 1971.

Amen, Daniel G., M.D. *Change Your Brain, Change Your Life.* New York: Three Rivers Press, 1998.

Amen, Daniel G., M.D. *Magnificent Mind at Any Age.* New York: Random House, Inc., 2008.

Ammon-Wexler, J., Ph.D. "An Investigation of the Influences of Visually-Perceived Colored Light Stimulation on Subjects with Phobic Disorders." Los Gatos, CA: Innerspace Biofeedback and Therapy Center, January, 1990.

Anderson, M.D. and J.M. Williams. *"Seeing Too Straight; Stress and Vision,"* Longevity, August, 1989.

Andreas, Steve, and Connirae Andreas. *Change Your Mind and Keep the Change.* Moab, UT: Real People Press, 1987.

Anshell, Jeffrey, O.D. *Healthy Eyes, Better Vision.* Los Angeles, CA: The Body Press, 1990.

Anshell, Jeffrey, O.D. *Smart Medicine for Your Eyes.* Garden City Park, NY: Avery Publishing Group, 1999.

Anshell, Jeffrey, O.D. *Visual Ergonomics in the Workplace.* Bristol, PA: Taylor and Francis, Inc., 1998.

Bandler, Richard, and John Grinder. *Frogs into Princes.* Moab, UT: Real People Press, 1979.

Bandler, Richard, and John Grinder. *Reframing.* Moab, UT: Real People Press, 1982.

Bandler, Richard, and John Grinder. *The Structure of Magic I and II.* Palo Alto, CA: Science and Behavior Books, Inc., 1975.

Bates, W. H., M.D. *Better Eyesight Without Glasses.* New York: Henry Holt and Company, 1920.

Bates, William H., M.D. *The Bates Method for Better Eyesight Without Glasses.* New York, NY: Pyramid Books, 1940.

Battenberg, Jane R. "The Effects of the Lumatron on Visual Field and Learning and Emotional Abilities." Fountain Valley, CA: unpublished paper, September, 1992.

Begley, Sharon. *Train Your Mind; Change Your Brain.* New York: Ballantine Books, Random House, Inc., 2007.

Beresford, Dr. Steven M., Dr. David W. Muirs, Dr. Merrill J. Allen, and Dr. Francis A. Young. *Improve Your Vision Without Glasses or Contact Lenses.* New York, NY: Simon and Schuster, 1996.

Berne, Samuel, O.D. *Creating Your Personal Vision.* Santa Fe, NM: Color Stone Press, 1994.

Blakeslee, Sandra. "Study Ties Dyslexia to Brain Flaw Affecting Vision and Other Senses." *New York Times.* Sunday, September 15, 1991.

Breiling, Brian, and Lee Hartley. *Light Years Ahead: The Illustrated Guide to Full Spectrum and Colored Light in Mindbody Healing.* Berkeley, CA: Celestial Arts, 1996.

Brown University. www.cog.brown.edu/courses/c0001/lectures/visualpaths.html.

Capra, Fritjof. *The Tao of Physics.* Boulder, CO: Shambhala Publications, 1975.

Cassel, Gary H., M.D., Michael D. Billig, O.D., and Harry G. Randall, M.D. *The Eye Book: A Complete Guide to Eye Disorders and Health.* Baltimore, MD: The Johns Hopkins University Press, 1998.

Chopra, Deepak, M.D. *Ageless Body, Timeless Mind.* New York, NY: Harmony Books, 1993.

Chopra, Deepak, M.D. *Perfect Health.* New York, NY: Harmony Books, 1991.

Cook, David L., O.D., FCOVD. *Vision: What Every Pilot Needs to Know.* Atlanta, GA: Invision Press, 1991.

Corbett, Margaret Darst. *Help Yourself to Better Sight.* Chatsworth, CA: Wilshire Book Company, 1995.

Crocco, John A., M.D. *Gray's Anatomy.* New York, NY: Bounty Books, 1977.

Csikszentmihalyi, Mihaly. *Flow: The Psychology of Optimal Experience.* New York, NY: Harper Perennial, 1990.

D'Alonzo, Dr. T.L., O.D. *Your Eyes! A Comprehensive Look at Understanding and Treatment of Vision Problems.* Clifton Heights, PA: Avanti Publishing, 1991.

Dallé, Suzan Wilkerson. Brochure for "Brain Integration Training," April, 1995.

Dallé, Suzan Wilkerson. Tapes of her workshop, *Brain Integration Training,* Bodega Bay, CA: August, 1993.

Deimel, Diana. *Vision Victory Via Vital Foods, Visual Training & Vitamins.* Fillmore, CA: Diana Deimel, 1972.

Delis-Abrams, Alexandra, Ph.D. *Improved Health Through Honoring Our Feelings.* http://www.theattitudedoc.com/resources/articles/health.

Dennison, Paul E., Ph.D. *Switching On: The Holistic Answer to Dyslexia.* Glendale, CA: Edu-Kinesthetics, Inc., 1981.

Diamond, M.C., Ph.D., A.B. Scheibel, M.D., and L.M. Elson, Ph.D. *The Human Brain Coloring Book.* Oakville, CA: Coloring Concepts, Inc., 1985.

Dilts, Robert B. *Changing Belief Systems with NLP.* Capitola, CA: Meta Publications, Inc., 1990.

Dilts, Robert Brian. *Roots of Neuro-Linguistic Programming.* Cupertino, CA: Meta Publications, 1983.

Dilts, Robert B., Todd Epstein, and Robert W. Dilts. *Tools for Dreamers.* Capitola, CA: Meta Publications, Inc., 1991.

Dinshah, Darius. *Let There Be Light.* Malaga, NJ: Dinshah Health Society, 1985.

Doidge, Norman, M.D. *The Brain That Changes Itself.* New York, NY: Penguin Group (USA) Inc., 2007.

Donaldson, Lee, and Jonathan Rand. *Pushing Up The Sky.* Crystal Lake, IL: Candlewick Press, 1997.

Eames, T. H. "Restrictions of the Visual Field as Handicaps to Learning." *Journal of Educational Research 19* (February, 1936): 460-463.

Eames, T. H. "The Relationship of the Central Vision Field to the Speed of Visual Perception." *American Journal of Ophthalmology,* 43 (1957): 279-289.

Eden, Donna. *Energy Medicine for Women: Aligning Your Body's Energies to Boost Your Health and Vitality.* London, England: Penguin Books Ltd., 2008.

Edwards, Betty. *The New Drawing on the Right Side of the Brain.* USA: Penguin Group Incorporated, August, 1999.

Eulenberg, Alexander. "The Case for the Preventability of Myopia." Bloomington, IN: March 3, 1996, 1-20. http://php.indiana.edu/~see/prevent_myopia.html.

Fitness Science Excerpted from Marilyn Roy's *EyeRobics©, 1999,* "Great Eyesight for the Rest of Your Life!" First for Women Magazine, October 25, 1999.

Forrest, Elliott B., O.D. *Visual Imagery: An Optometric Approach.* Duncan, OK: Optometric Extension Program Foundation, Inc., 1981.

Gallop, Steve, O.D. "Myopia Reduction – A View From the Inside." *Journal of Behavioral Optometry* Volume 5, Number 5 (1994): 115-120.

Gallop, Steve, O.D. "What's So Great About 20/20? Or… The Plight of Nearsightedly-challenged Individuals." *Journal of Behavioral Optometry* Number 2, Volume 12 (1994): 41-46.

Gerard, R. M. "Differential Effects of Colored Lights on Psycho-physiological Functions." University of California, Los Angeles, psychology dissertation (1958).

Gerber, Richard. *Vibrational Medicine.* Santa Fe, NM: Bear and Company, 1954.

Glicksman, Dr. Howard. Exercise Your Wonder with Dr. G. "Wired for Much More than Sound: Part IV: Vision Part 1—Parts of the Eye." http://www.arn.org/docs/glicksman/eyw_041001.htm.

Glicksman, Dr. Howard. Vision Part 3 — *What Does the Brain See?* http://www.arn.org/docs/glicksman/eyw_041201.htm. "Wired for Much More than Sound: Part VI: Vision Part 3—What Does the Brain See?

Goodrich, Janet, Ph.D. *Help Your Child to Perfect Eyesight Without Glasses.* Berkeley, CA: Celestial Arts, 1996.

Goodrich, Janet, Ph.D. *Natural Vision Improvement.* Berkeley, CA: Celestial Arts, 1985.

Goodwin, Dr. Paul. *Foundation Theory: Report on the Efficacy of the Formal Education Process in Rural Alaska, Volume 1.* Honolulu, HI: Advanced Neuro Dynamics, Inc., 1988.

Gordon, David. *Therapeutic Metaphors.* Capitola, CA: Meta Publications, 1978.

Gottlieb, Raymond L., O.D., Oh.D. "Neuropsychology of Myopia," excerpted from Doctoral Dissertation. *Journal of Optometric Vision Development,* Volume XIII, Number 1 (March, 1982): 3-27.

Gray, Henry, F.R.S. *Gray's Anatomy: The Classic Collectors' Edition.* U.S.A.: Bounty Books, 1977.

Gregory, R.L. *Eye and the Brain.* New York: McGraw Hill, 1966.

Grinder, John and Richard Bandler. *Trance-formations: Neuro-Linguistic Programming and the Structure of Hypnosis.* Moab, UT: Real People Press, 1981.

Grossman, Marc, O.D., L.Ac, and Vinton McCabe. *Greater Vision —A Guide to Physical, Emotional and Spiritual Clarity in Everyday Life.* McGraw Hill, 2001.

Grossman, Marc, O.D., L.Ac. and Glen Swartwout, O.D. *Natural Eye Care: An Encyclopedia.* Los Angeles, CA: Keats Publishing, 1999.

Hampden-Turner, Charles. *Maps of the Mind.* New York: MacMillan Publishing Co., Inc., 1981.

Hay, Louise L. *Heal Your Body: The Mental Causes for Physical Illness and the Metaphysical Way to Overcome Them.* Santa Monica, CA: Hay House, 1982.

Henning, W. "The Fundamentals of Chrome-Orthoptics." Chicago, IL: Actino Laboratories, Inc., 1936.

Hollwich, E. *The Influence of Ocular Light Perception on Metabolisms in Man and in Animal.* New York, NY: Springer-Verlag, 1979.

Houston, Dr. Jean. *Jump Time.* New York, NY: Jeremy P. Tarcher/Putnam, 2000.

Houston, Dr. Jean. *The Possible Human.* New York, NY: Jeremy P. Tarcher/Putnam, 2002.

Houston, Dr. Jean. *The Search for the Beloved.* New York, NY: St. Martin's Press, 1987.

http://www.cog.brown.edu/courses/cg0001/lectures/visual-paths.html. (Notes on visual pathways to brain hemispheres).

http://www.paulapeterson.com/Living_On_Light.html (Quotes on sunlight under Sunning). (Source for Wilma Rudolph quote.)

Hubel, David. *Eye, Brain and Vision.* http://neuro.med.harvard.edu/site/dh/bcontex.htm: July, 1995.

Hutchison, Michael. *Megabrain: New Tools and Techniques for Brain Growth and Mind Expansion.* New York: Ballantine Books, 1986.

Huxley, Aldous L. *The Art of Seeing.* Seattle, WA: Montana Books, 1975 (reissue of original 1942 version).

James, Tad and Wyatt Woodsmall. *Time Line Therapy and the Basis of Personality.* Capitola, CA: Meta Publications, 1988.

Jensen, Bernard, D.C. *The Science and Practice of Iridology.* Escondido, CA: Bernard Jensen, 1974.

Johnson, Denny Ray, with J. Erik Ness. *What The Eye Reveals.* Boulder, CO: Rayid Publications, 1995.

Kaplan, R. "Changes in Form Visual Fields in Reading Disabled Children Produced by Syntonic Stimulation." *International Journal of Biosocial Research,* 5 Number 1 (1983): 20-33.

Kaplan, Robert Michael, O.D. *Conscious Seeing.* Hillsboro, OR: Beyond Words Publishing, 2002.

Kaplan, R. M. "Light, Lenses and The Mind—The Potent Medicine of Optometry." *Journal of Optometric Vision Development,* 4 (Autumn, 2002): 153-160.

Kaplan, Roberto M., O.D., M.Ed., FCOVD. "Nearsightedness: Seeing Beyond The Obvious." *Journal of Optometric Vision Development,* 14, (Summer, 2003): 64-70.

Kaplan, Robert Michael, O.D. *Seeing Without Glasses: Improving Your Vision Naturally.* Hillsboro, OR: Beyond Words Publishing, 1994.

Kaplan, Robert Michael. "The Art of Seeing: The Vision Alternatives Approach of Robert-Michael Kaplan." *East West Magazine* (December, 1986): 40-45.

Kaplan, Robert Michael, O.D. *The Power Behind Your Eyes.* Rochester, VT: Healing Arts Press, 1995.

Kavner, Richard S., O.D., and Lorraine Dusky. *Total Vision.* Millwood, NY: Kavner Books, 1978.

Keirsey, David, and Marilyn Bates. *Please Understand Me—Character and Temperament Types.* Essex, United Kingdom: Prometheus, 1978.

Kirby, Dale. *Meta-Web—NLP Mega-Glossary.* http://www.rain. org/~dale/nlpgloss.html.

Kondrot, Edward, and Edward C. Coors, M.D. *Healing the Eye the Natural Way.* Berkeley, CA: North Atlantic Books, 2001.

Lavery, Michael J. *Whole Brain Power: The Fountain of Youth for the Mind and Body.* Blaine, WA: LULU Print on Demand, September, 2008.

Leviton, R. *Seven Steps to Better Vision.* Brookline, MA: East/West Natural Health Books, 1992.

Lewin, Roger. "Is Your Brain Really Necessary?" *Science 210* (new series) no. 4475 (December 12, 1980): 1232-1234.

Lewis, Byron, and Frank Pucelik. *The Magic of NLP Demystified.* London, United Kingdom: Specialist Publications, 1985.

Liberman, Jacob, O.D., Ph.D. *Light: Medicine of the Future.* Santa Fe, NM: Bear and Company Publishing, 1991.

Liberman, Jacob, O.D., Ph.D. *Take Off Your Glasses and See: A Mind/Body Approach to Expanding Your Eyesight and Insight.* New York, NY: Crown Publishing, 1995.

Liberman, Jacob. *Wisdom from an Empty Mind.* Empty Mind Publications, April, 2001.

Lipton, Bruce. *The Biology of Belief.* Santa Rosa, CA: Mountains of Love/Elite Books, 2005.

Lofting, C.J. "Hemispheres of the Brain as Objects (What)/Relationships (Where) Processors. http://pages.prodigy.net/lofting/hemis.html: copyright 1995-2003.

Mansfield, Peter. *The Bates Method: A Complete Guide to Improving Eyesight—Naturally.* London, England: Random House, 1996.

Marsh, Doug. *Restoring Your Eyesight: A Taoist Approach.* Rochester, VT: Healing Arts Press, 2007.

Meluso, John Jr. *eye Talk*™. Carmel, CA: Positive Living, Inc., 2001.

Orfield, Antonia, M.A., O.D. "Seeing Space: Undergoing Brain Re-Programming to Reduce Myopia." *Journal of Behavioral Optometry,* Volume 5, Number 5 (1994): 123-131.

Ornstein, Robert E. *The Psychology of Consciousness.* New York: Harcourt Brace Jovanovich, Inc., 1977.

Penfield, Wilder, M.D., and Theodore Rasmussen. *The Cerebral Cortex of Man.* New York: Macmillan, 1950.

Pert, Candace B. *Molecules of Emotion.* New York, NY: Scribner, 1997.

Ponte, L. "How Color Affects Your Moods and Health." *Readers Digest* (July, 1982).

Ponte, L. "Light Can Improve IQs of Children." *Southland News* (Sunday, June 20, 1982).

Quackenbush, Thomas. *Better Eyesight: The Complete Magazines of William H. Bates.* Berkeley, CA: North Atlantic Books, 2001.

Quackenbush, Thomas R. *Relearning to See.* Berkeley, CA: North Atlantic Books, 1997.

Ramachandran, V. S., M.D., Ph.D., and Sandra Blakeslee. *Phantoms in the Brain: Probing the Mysteries of the Human Mind.* New York, NY: HarperCollins Publishers, Inc., 1998.

Robertson, Raye. "The Single Eye." *The Mountain Astrologer* (April/May, 2006): 23-59.

Rosanes-Berrett, Marilyn. *Do You Really Need Eyeglasses?* New York: Station Hill Press, 1990.

Rose, Marc R., M.D., and Michael R. Rose, M.D. *Save Your Sight! Natural Ways to Prevent and Reverse Macular Degeneration.* New York, NY: Time Warner Company, 1998.

Rotté, Joanna, Ph.D., and Koji Yamamoto. *Vision: A Holistic Guide to Healing the Eyesight.* Tokyo, Japan, and New York, NY: Japan Publications, Inc., 1985.

Rustigan, C. J. "The Effects of Colored Lights and Relaxation Exercises on Learning Disabled Adults' Visual and Learning Skills." Sacramento, CA: California State University, unpublished paper (December, 1991).

Samuels, Mike, M.D., and Nancy Samuels. *Seeing With The Mind's Eye.* New York, NY: Random House, Inc., and La Jolla, CA: The Bookworks, 1975.

Schiffer, Frederic, M.D. http://www.schiffermd.com.

Schiffer, Frederic, M.D. *Two Minds: The Revolutionary Science of Dual-Brain Psychology.* New York: The Free Press, 1998.

Schneider, Meir. *Self-Healing: My Life and Vision.* London, England: Routledge and Kegan, Penguin Group, 1987.

Schneider, Meir, and Maureen Larkin. *The Handbook of Self-Healing.* New York, NY: Penguin Books, 1994.

Scholl, Lisette. *28 Days to Reading Without Glasses.* Secaucus, NJ: Citadel Press Books, 1998.

Scholl, Lisette. *Visionetics: The Holistic Way to Better Eyesight.* Garden City, NY: Doubleday, 1978.

Schwartz, Jeffrey M., M.D., and Sharon Begley. *The Mind and the Brain: Neuroplasticity and the Power of Mental Force.* New York, NY: HarperCollins Publishers, 2002.

Sheldrake, Rupert. *A New Science of Life.* Rochester, VT: Park Street Press, 1981.

Shlain, Leonard. *The Alphabet Versus the Goddess: The Conflict Between Word and The Image.* New York: Penguin Compass, 1998.

Simonton, O. Carl, Stephanie Matthews-Simonton, and James L. Creighton. *Getting Well Again.* New York: Scientific American Library, 1996.

Sussman, Martin, and Ernest Liewenstein. *Total Health at the Computer.* Barrytown, NY: Station Hill Press, 1993.

Sussman, Martin. *The Program for Better Vision.* Topsfield, MA: K-See Publications, 1985.

Talbot, Michael. *The Holographic Universe.* New York, NY: Harper Collins Publishers, 1991.

Tortora, Gerard J., and Sandra Reynolds Grabowski. *Principles of Anatomy and Physiology.* New York, NY: John Wiley and Sons, Inc., 2003.

Wake, Lisa. *Neurolinguistic Psychotherapy: A Postmodern Approach.* London: Routledge, 2008. www.awakenconsulting.co.uk.

Wexler, B.E. *Brain and Culture: Neurobiology, Ideology and Social Change.* Cambridge, MA: MIT Press, 2006.

Woolf, V. Vernon, Ph.D. *Holodynamics: How to Develop and Manage Your Personal Power.* Tucson and New York: Harbinger House, 1990.

Zajonc, Arthur. *Catching the Light: The Entwined History of Light and Mind.* New York, NY: Bantam Books, 1993.

Zukav, Gary. *The Dancing Wu Li Masters.* Toronto and New York: Bantam Books, 1979.

INDEX

20/20 – 148, 156, 199, 200, 298

A

accommodation, 166, 294, 295, 296
ADD (Attention Deficit Disorder), 131
aiming, 62, 71, 73, 85, 192
Alexander Technique, 169, 287
Ammon-Wexler, Jill, 186, 299
analytical, 51, 53-54, 81, 89, 90, 100, 102, 128-129, 149, 204, 245, 272, 296
ancestral, 215-216
Andreas, Steve and Connirae, 223, 299
anger, 145, 150, 160-161, 164, 185, 191, 228, 234-235, 245
Apple, Neal, ii, 119, 283
astigmatism, 32, 91, 143, 145, 151, 153, 163-165, 168-169, 196, 286, 294
attention, 19, 34, 47, 58, 59-61, 77, 78, 81, 87, 97, 112, 122, 138, 159, 160, 183, 185, 186, 189-191, 192, 196, 206, 217-218, 224, 226, 247, 272, 278, 279, 294
auditory, 19-24, 27-28, 33, 35, 37, 105, 126-129, 131, 133, 165, 185, 272, 275, 276, 295, 296, 298
auditory-digital, 128, 272, 276
autonomic nervous system (ANS), 103, 113, 122, 183, 253

B

Bach-y-Rita, Paul, 40
balance
    brain functions, 50, 53, 82, 105,186
    logical and emotional, 54, 82, 127, 186
    physical, 35, 36, 38, 127, 137, 158, 168
Bandler, Richard, 19, 24, 276, 296, 300, 304
Bates Method, 9, 11, 169, 282, 285, 294, 300, 307
Bates, William H., x, 11, 93, 94, 95, 114, 156, 179, 180, 181, 294, 300, 307
Battenberg, Jane, xvii, xviii, xxii, xxiv, 37, 83, 157, 162, 176-177, 181, 201, 221, 246, 292, 300
behavioral optometry, 284, 291, 294, 298
beliefs
    about vision, 103, 104, 138, 164, 198, 199, 211, 223, 226, 279
    limiting, about eyesight, xxv, 103, 104, 211, 216, 219, 227, 229, 237, 298
    shape reality,138, 223-224, 226
Berne, Sam, i, xix, 8, 167-168, 283-284, 300
bilateral integration, 167, 168
binocular vision, 294
Blakeslee, Sandra, 184, 300, 308

Brown University, 117, 300, 305
blind spot, 37-38, 90, 183, 186, 187
blinking, 11-12, 203, 242, 256, 260
Bohm, David, 223, 230
brain
    changed by learning, 148
    changed by therapy, 230, 238
    deletes, distorts, generalizes information, 138, 224, 226, 279
    eye-brain connection, x, xix, 10, 17, 45, 51, 82, 99, 164, 238, 255
    internal representations (functions), 19, 27, 223-227, 238, 296, 298
    memory, (see memory)
    neuroplasticity, plasticity of, 40, 180, 206-207, 227-228, 230
    rapport with eyes, 80, 84, 89, 219, 238
    right brain, left brain functions, 45-53, 82, 89, 100, 105
    structures of, 49, 148, 159
    shuts down vision, 56, 80-82, 164
    tells the eyes to turn on sight, 79, 84, 99
    turns on sight, 79, 83-84, 99
breathing, xxii, 31, 32, 98, 156, 171, 203, 242, 252, 254, 275, 276

C

Cass, Elizabeth, 171, 311
cataract(s), 151, 196, 204, 296
central vision, 113, 116, 156, 158, 295
Chopra, Deepak, 228-229, 301

ciliary muscles, 111, 113, 161, 202, 294, 295
circadian rhythm, 121
circle, closer, 67, 68, 249
circles, 3-D effect, 67, 83, 90
clairvoyance, 198
clear sight, split instances of, 80, 179, 259
Clock Circles, 15-17, 20, 26, 27, 30, 32, 35, 37, 243
close work, 11, 113, 155, 167, 171, 199, 201, 242, 260
color blind, 201, 204, 220
combinatory play, 48
computer(s), ix, xi, 47, 112, 155, 199
computer games, 206
computer work, 91, 158, 162, 169, 172, 193, 202, 203
concentration, 81, 162, 167, 168, 171, 183, 186, 189, 191, 198
cones, 92, 113, 120, 295
conscious awareness, 47
conscious mind, 103, 233, 234, 236
converge, convergence, 55, 60, 62, 65-66, 68, 70-72, 248-249, 295
converging, 42, 68, 110
Cook, David L., 122, 301
cool down, xxiv, 8, 91, 252, 258
cornea, 32, 91, 110-111, 115, 116, 145, 163-164, 201, 295, 296
corpus callosum, 47, 50, 295
corrective lens(es), 104, 144, 164
creativity, 21, 27, 46, 49, 53, 175, 195, 253, 279, 298
critical flicker fusion, 188
cross crawl, 13, 37, 166, 167, 242, 256
Csikszentmihalyi, Mihaly, 224, 226, 280, 301

D

da Vinci, Leonardo, 41, 297
daily Eye Yoga, xxiii, 10, 28, 55, 84, 99
Dale, Theresa, 230
Dallé, Suzan Wilkerson, xix, 118, 143, 179-180, 301
Deimel, Diana, 126, 301
Delis-Abrams, Alexandra, 230, 301
depression, 157, 186, 235, 245, 284
depth perception, 47, 56-57, 83, 115-116, 161, 184, 192, 220, 247, 294
digital (auditory-digital), 23, 128, 272, 276
Dilts, Robert, 22, 302
dissociated, 25
Doidge, Norman, 40, 180, 206, 207, 208-230, 302
dominant eye, 50, 79, 99, 102
dopamine, 206
double vision, 56, 77, 201, 247
Downing, John, 186
dyslexia, 25, 167, 168, 184

E

Eames, T. H., 302
Edelman, George, 229
Edwards, Betty, 53, 302
Einstein, Albert, 48
EMDR (Eye Movement Desensitization Response), 22, 284
emotional stability, 186
emotional trauma, 150
emotions, 21, 25, 45, 46, 52, 101-102, 119, 122, 127, 130, 139, 143, 147, 148, 149, 151, 152, 155, 158, 160, 161, 164-165, 168, 179, 185, 196, 197, 214, 216-219, 220-221, 226, 228, 229, 230, 234, 236-238, 245, 251, 272, 278, 292, 296, 298
Eskimo(s), 171, 174
Eulenberg, Alexander, 152-153, 156, 171, 174, 302
eye-accessing patterns, 25, 295
eye(s)
  aim(ing), 57-58, 60, 62, 66, 70-71, 73-74, 85, 87, 192
  as extension of the brain, 109, 139, 144
  cross(ed), 42, 59-60, 65-66, 73, 160, 201, 247, 248
  decision to limit sight, 215, 218
  dominant, 50, 53, 79, 82, 99, 102
  flexibility, 9, 18, 42, 57, 73, 91, 147-148, 150, 156, 162, 172, 196
  hardwired into the brain, 40, 139, 143, 183
  movement, 10, 12, 16, 17-18, 20-21, 22, 24, 26-27, 33, 44, 57, 113, 114, 115, 153, 168, 185
  muscles, 9-10, 11, 15, 32, 45, 57, 81, 91, 96, 98, 110-111, 113-114, 156, 161, 163, 181, 202, 220, 251, 255, 295,
  nasal image, 117-120
  patch, 51, 101, 251
  patching, 50, 51, 99-105, 120, 250-251, 257-258
  physiology of, 110-114
  precision, 57, 73
  relation to spatial orientation, 156
  see together, 9, 79, 294
  strain, ix, 15, 45, 91, 94, 96, 156, 162, 180, 258
  temporal image, 117, 118, 119
  unique personality of each eye, 51, 100, 118-119, 137

F

farsighted, 71, 85, 91, 114, 143-147, 150, 152, 160-161, 163, 196, 295
fear, 21, 91, 102, 143, 144, 149-150, 154-155, 158, 164, 196, 213, 228, 232-235, 245
field of vision, 16, 183, 186
Figure 8, 30-37, 63, 68, 69, 244, 248, 259
Finger Push-Ups, 42-45, 53-55, 244, 259
Fleming, Tony, 38-40
flicker rate, 186, 188
floaters, 196
fovea, 113, 137, 158, 295, 296
foveal vision, 137

G

Galin, David, 82
Gallop, Steven, 153-154, 158-159, 172-173, 200, 303
games, computer, 206
ganglion cells, 111, 120
Gardiner, P. A., 171
Gerard, R. M., 184-185, 303
Glas, Alan, 38
glaucoma, 196, 284
Glicksman, Howard, 303
glitches, 16-17, 20, 28, 44, 54, 245
Goodrich, Janet, 286, 287, 303
Goodwin, Paul, 229, 303
Gottlieb, Ray, i, xix, 160, 282, 304
Gray, Henry, 109, 301, 304
Grinder, John, 19, 24, 276, 296, 300, 304
Grossman, Marc, 202, 282, 304
guilt, 228

H

hand-eye coordination, 41, 132, 167, 168
haptic, 128, 131, 135
Harris, Paul, 169
Hay, Louise, 198, 304
head tilt, 17, 55, 71
Henning, W., 183, 304
holistic, 46, 51, 53-54, 92, 100, 144, 151, 167
holographic, 38, 223-231
hormones, 121, 138, 228, 297
Houston, Jean, i, xix, 35, 177, 178, 229, 288-289, 304-305
Hunt, R., 34
Hutchison, Michael, 185, 305
hyperactivity, 185-186
hypnosis, 39, 123, 253, 284

I

imagination, 39, 46, 49, 87, 177, 179, 180, 198, 227, 229, 236, 253-254
immune system, 177, 235
inner mind, 164
insight, i, xxi, xxii, 10, 21, 26, 81, 82, 136, 146, 148, 180, 191, 195, 197, 203, 212, 217, 220, 232, 237, 264, 293
internal representation, 19, 27, 223-227, 238, 272-273, 275, 276, 295, 296, 298
intuitive, xiii 46, 53, 83, 101, 126, 130 180, 298
IQ, 144, 184, 231, 307
iridology, 125-126
iris
    analysis, 136
    blueprint of inheritance, 126
    emotional traits seen in, 126
    Flower, 127

innate personality seen in,
126-128, 139
Jewel, 127
Shaker, 127, 128
Stream, 127
structures, 127

J

James, Tad, xix, 276, 277, 280, 305
James, William, 122
Jensen, Bernard, 126, 305
Johnson, Denny Ray, 126-128,
136, 305
Josephson, Emanuel, 171
journal(ing), 41, 101, 245-246,
251
Jump Vs, 62-64, 248
movement variations, 63
troubleshooting, 63
jumps, 16-17, 20, 28, 44, 54, 244
Circle Jumps, 70, 249
saccades, 121

K

Kandel, Eric, 147, 159, 230
Kaplan, Roberto, xviii, xix, 42, 119,
127, 136, 144, 146, 154-155,
160-161, 164, 169, 170, 173,
185, 198, 285, 287-288,
305-306
Keats, John, 143
Keirsey-Bates (Keirsey, David, and
Marilyn Bates), 277, 280, 306
kinesthetic, 19-20, 23, 25-28, 33-35,
46, 105, 126-131, 134, 177, 180,
272, 276, 295, 296, 298
Kirby, Dale, 18, 306
Knots on a String, 63, 65, 73-78,
83, 93, 249-250
seeing only one string, 75, 80,

81, 83, 85-89
seeing two strings, 74, 77-82,
84-86, 88-89
Kondrot, Edward, 284, 306

L

Lane, Ben, 170
lateral geniculate nucleus (LGN),
120-121
Lavery, Michael, 41, 306
left brain, 11, 13, 35, 45-52, 53,
81, 82-84, 89-90, 99-102, 105,
117-120, 126, 136, 138, 238,
242, 245, 296
left eye/right brain, 89, 100, 204
left hemisphere, 45, 117-118, 296
lens (eye part), 110-111, 113, 116,
145, 162, 163-164, 201-202,
294-297
lens (prescription), 101, 104, 144,
147, 148, 153-159, 161-162,
171-173, 195, 202-203, 260,
288, 296, 297
Lewin, Roger, 231, 306
Liberman, Jacob, i, xix, 50, 80,
111, 114, 115, 122, 139, 144,
145, 170, 185, 192, 211, 284,
306-307
lifeline, 216, 218, 233, 235, 237
light as a nutrient, 92, 95, 183, 186,
251
light sensitivity, xiii, 92, 97
light, colored, as therapy, xii-xiii,
104, 183-186, 188, 192, 299,
300, 303, 308
logical, 51-54, 81, 82, 89-90, 100,
101, 102, 119, 155, 198, 245,
251, 277, 278
Lumatron, xiii, 185-186, 188,
191-192, 300

M

macular degeneration, 170, 196, 284, 308

magnocellular, 184

McLuhan, Marshall, 205-206

Mead, Margaret, 21-22

media, electronic, 206

meditation, 50, 99, 220

Meluso, John, 128, 136, 307

memorizing, 24, 49, 275, 276

memory, 18, 24, 49, 168, 171, 175, 179, 180, 183, 185, 186, 189, 190, 217, 223, 227

Mendelsohn, Celeste, xix, 110, 111, 114, 118, 132-135, 225

mental facility, 27

mental strain, 155, 156, 181, 202

Merzenich, Michael, 40

metaprograms, 277, 279,280

Meyers, Ronald, 47

mirror-image writing, 41

model of reality, 224, 225

model of the world, 224

multiple personalities, 147, 229

Multiple Personality Disorder (MPD), 147, 229, 230

Myers-Briggs, 272, 277, 280

myopia, i, 85, 91, 149-150, 151-159, 171, 173, 181, 202-203, 282, 296, 302, 303, 304, 307

myopic, 119, 153-154, 171, 173, 202-203, 296

N

Nazmy, Mohamed, 35-36

nearsighted, nearsightedness, 6, 72, 85, 91, 114, 143, 144, 145, 146, 147, 149-150, 151-159, 160, 161, 163, 166, 170, 171, 172, 173, 174, 181, 196, 202-203, 267, 286, 296, 303, 305

neural circuits, 229

Neuro-Linguistic Programming, see NLP

neurons, 41, 121, 207, 223, 229, 230, 297

NLP, xiii, xxiii, 18, 19, 21, 22, 25, 33, 34, 128, 165, 222, 223, 224, 276, 296, 297, 302, 306

NLP model of reality, 224, 225

Nobel Prize, 47, 147, 230

O

occipital bone, 93

optic chiasm, 47

optic nerve, xvii, 92, 94, 109-110, 111, 120, 121, 137, 186, 187, 251, 298

Optician, 104, 297

optics, 104, 153

Optometrist, x, xi, xii , 8, 104, 119, 144, 157, 163, 164, 167, 169, 170, 173, 179, 192, 281, 282, 288, 289, 290, 291, 297, 298

Orfield, Antonia, 147, 156, 157, 166, 173, 307

Ornstein, Robert, 48, 82, 123, 307

P

palming, 28, 54, 60-61, 67-68, 69, 71, 82, 91-94, 97, 98, 167, 244, 247, 248, 249, 251, 252, 254, 256, 257, 258, 259

panoramic, 73

Pascual-Leone, Alvaro, 174

past life, 120, 214-216, 235

patching, 50, 51, 99-102, 105, 120, 250-251, 257

Peczely, Ignatz von, 125

Penfield, Wilder, 123, 307
peripheral color distinction, 187-188
peripheral vision, 37, 66, 78, 101, 113, 137, 153, 156, 158-159, 162, 168, 180, 186, 188, 190, 259
Pert, Candace, 228, 307
pinhole glasses, 297
pituitary, 122
postural training, 166, 168-169
posture, 17, 84, 148, 151, 163, 166, 168-169, 250, 260, 294
presbyopia, 55, 85, 91, 145, 150, 161-162, 196, 282, 297
prescription strength, 147, 148, 153, 154, 155, 156, 158, 171-173, 202, 220
Pribram, Karl, 123, 223, 230
psychic abilities, 198
pupil, 12, 97-98, 110, 121, 125, 138, 252, 295, 296

R

rapport, 80, 84, 89, 103, 130, 146-147, 219, 238, 273
Rayid Method, 127, 305
Representational System(s), (see internal representation)
retinal detachment, 196, 220
retinal discrimination, 112
rhythm, circadian, 121
right brain, 45-54, 81, 82, 83, 89, 90, 99, 100, 101, 102, 117-119, 126, 138, 204, 251, 298
right eye/left brain, 51-53, 81-83, 89-90
right hemisphere, 45, 48, 117, 175
Rigney, Martha, vii, xvii-xviii, xxiv, 181, 193, 201, 221, 283

ritalin, 185
Robertson, Raye, 199, 308
rods, 92, 113, 120, 221
Rose, Marc R. and Michael R., 170, 308
rotations, head and neck, 13, 167, 242
Rotté, Joanna, 92, 205, 308
Rubin, Peggy, 35

S

saccades, 121
sadness, 25, 176, 196, 228, 235
Scholl, Lisette, 200, 308
Seasonal Affective Disorder (SAD), 284
Schiffer, Fred, 48, 120, 308
Shlain, Leonard, 49, 309
sclera, 110-111, 125
second sight, 198
SEE Circles, 14, 65-71, 73, 248-249
SEE Circles, clear plastic squares, 72, 249, 270
SEE clear, 66, 67, 69, 70
see clearly, xvii, 80, 147, 154, 162, 179, 211, 213, 219, 259, 295
See In, 70, 71, 248-249
See Out, 68, 70, 71, 72, 249
seeing double, 56, 77, 201, 115, 247
self hypnosis, 39, 253
sets of circles, 65-67, 68-71, 249
Sheldrake, Rupert, 230, 309
short-arm syndrome, 55, 161-162
sight, as a metaphor, 148, 154, 194-197, 198, 205, 212, 213, 220
Sikes, Rex Steven, 17, 18
Simonton, O. Carl and Stephanie

Matthews, 175, 309

Sinclair, J., 32

sounds, 11, 19, 20, 21, 22-26, 32, 33, 46, 115, 126, 179, 213, 223, 224-226, 232-233, 242, 272, 273, 274, 296

spatial, 51, 53, 82, 116, 137, 156, 158, 260
awareness, 46, 113, 137, 152, 156
discrimination, 112
distortion, 153, 156

Sperry, Roger, 47-48, 50-51

Spinelli, 123

spiritual(ity), 37, 126, 148, 162, 197, 198, 292

staring, 11, 20, 34, 77, 242, 260

strategies, 21, 23-24, 46

stress, 37, 76, 81, 82, 84, 85, 89, 91, 147, 148, 150, 156, 158, 159, 170, 172, 180-182, 184, 185, 186, 189, 190, 203, 205, 211, 213, 253, 284, 293, 294, 298

stress reduction, 186, 189

stress, mental, 211, 294

stress, emotional, 91, 180, 205, 211, 294

stroke, 32, 33-41, 176, 206, 207, 231

sunglasses, 97, 101

Sunning, 91, 92, 95, 96, 97, 98, 251, 252, 257, 258, 259

Sunning, flicker variation, 97, 252, 260

suppression, 56, 63, 74, 81, 83, 85, 88, 89, 90, 99, 113, 116, 119, 123, 150, 161, 298

Sussman, Martin, 200, 283, 309

synaptic connections, 229, 230, 297

synesthesia, 21

Syntonic, 183, 186, 192, 282

T

Talbot, Michael, 223, 231, 309

team teaching both eyes, 56

teaming, 74, 192

tennis ball on a string, 29

Thiel, Peter Johannes, 126

Thomas, John, 173

Time Dimension Therapy (TDT), xiii, xix, 212, 213, 219, 220, 222-232, 233, 235, 238, 292, 298

Time Line Therapy©, 25, 280, 292, 305

traumatic event, 211, 217, 218

trombone, 63, 67, 69, 244, 248

TV, television, 49, 112, 172, 199, 206, 257, 297

Twist and Swing, 12, 242, 259

U

unconscious mind, 90, 103, 147, 158, 212, 214-216, 218-219, 232-238, 253, 298

V

values, 144, 145, 224, 226, 279, 280

V-In, 56, 59, 60, 61, 62, 71, 74, 247, 248, 249, 259

vision
and nutrition, 148, 159, 170-171, 196, 197, 258, 260, 284, 294
binocular, 86, 294, 298
central, 113, 116, 137, 156, 158, 295, 302
check, 3, 28, 54, 103, 254
clarity, 56, 81, 147, 179, 221, 259
connection with emotional conditions, 138, 147, 186,

211
context-dependent, 147
daydreaming, 123
double, 56, 77, 201, 247
eye-to-brain process, 119
fitness, 144
flexibility, 147-148, 156
foveal, 137
how we see, 84, 113, 144, 164, 199, 201, 264
inner, 144, 252
metaphor, 37, 148, 154, 194-199, 205, 212-213, 220
myths, i, 162, 199-200
peripheral, 37, 66, 78, 101, 113, 137, 153, 156, 158-159, 162, 166, 168, 180, 186, 187-188, 190, 259, 260
re-check, 3, 28, 54, 103, 254
shut down, 52, 53, 56, 63, 79-81, 82-83, 89, 90, 101, 164
switch off and on, 115
therapy, x, xii, 104, 119, 144, 155, 184-185, 282, 288, 289-290, 291, 294, 297, 298
three-dimensional, 83, 100
turn off in one eye, 89
two-dimensional, 83
visionaries, 198
visionary, i, 148, 198-199, 289
Visual Construct, 19, 22-24, 25-27, 35, 37, 121-123

visual cortex, 121, 138, 224
visual field, 117, 119, 156, 160, 183-187
Visual Remembered, 26, 33-34, 35, 37, 211
visual stimulation, 48
visualization(s), 32, 34-35, 37, 103, 123 168, 174-176, 177, 179, 198, 222, 233, 246, 252-253, 294, 298
V-Out, 56-57, 60, 61, 62, 71, 73, 74, 247, 248, 249, 259

W
Wake, Lisa, 25-26, 309
war of the brains, 48
Wexler, Bruce, 223, 227-228, 309
Whitehead, Alfred North, 124
whole brain, 49, 231, 306
wiggles, 16-17, 20, 26-28, 30, 44
womb, 215-216, 220, 235

Y
Yamamoto, Koji, 205, 308
yoga connection, xxiv
yoga exercises, 4, 10, 14, 28, 54, 162, 172, 253, 255, 259
yoga routine, xxi, 28, 241, 242
yoga, traditional, xxii

Z
zips, 16-17, 20, 26-28, 30